Praise for the POWER Eatir

"I found the initial seminar ⋯ ng about foods
that I the ⋯ ull of sugar i.e.
low fat y(⋯ ⋯ for my
energy le ⋯ ⋯ t 5 ⋯ n weight
in 4 weeks, although this was not my main goal. I'm sleeping
better too.

I feel good about myself now, eating more healthily and hope to
continue to boost my retirement years which are fast
approaching! I just need to cut the coffee down even more and
drink herbal teas (which I have discovered with this
programme).

I have really enjoyed doing this programme and will continue to
eat this way in the future. Thank you for introducing me to your
POWER Eating Programme™."

– Celia M. Accounts Manager

"I very nearly didn't make the effort to attend the presentation ...
but luckily I did and my eating habits have been changed for
good! I never ate breakfast, usually ate fruit for lunch and more
often than not ate the wrong things before my evening meal,
making me feel guilty as I'm always trying to lose weight.

This POWER Eating Programme™ does not feel like a diet, in fact
I'm eating much more than normal and don't feel hungry. I've
even lost 11 lbs and feel so much better. Many thanks, I know I
will never go back to my coffee, diet coke and low-fat lifestyle!"

– Loraine B. Administrator

"I have really enjoyed the experience. I found the food to be
satisfying and it felt good to be eating those lovely healthy foods
that I'd always avoided because of their high calorific values and
fat content. Happy to have lost 5lbs too. With all the nuts and
seeds there is no danger of constipation either! A real plus is that
it hasn't been a problem adapting the programme for the whole

family, I just cook the food we normally eat - meat, chicken, fish - but include lots more veg."

– Barbara B. Lettings Negotiator

"I always thought I was very aware of my diet but had no idea that the 'low-fat' options contained so much sugar! What an eye opener! I have really enjoyed the programme, lost 4 lbs and I definitely have more energy and sleep better. I intend to continue following the programme and look forward to experimenting with more meals. Many thanks."

– Maureen O. Lettings Negotiator

Since starting the POWER Eating Programme™ my energy levels do seem to be up and even after my cycle ride home I am full of beans! In the last 4 weeks I have lost nearly 5 kg and I'm very impressed with the success of the programme. I am continuing the healthy eating regime because I do actually enjoy it and find it very beneficial.

Having a food diary encouraged me to eat well because I would have felt naughty or embarrassed to put too many bad foods on it! However, I wanted it to be an honest reflection and if I did have a takeaway or something greasy I would still include it, as the programme needs to be realistic in order not to get bored and revert to previous habits.

One of the biggest revelations of the programme was learning about the hazards of "fat-free" alternatives. I now try to eat pure and natural products with minimal "tampering" wherever possible. This has been an enjoyable and enlightening experience.

– Matt E. Sales Support Administrator

No Caffeine Required

What to eat to energise your working day, naturally

Linda Munster

Email: **Linda@nocaffeinerequired.com**

Facebook: **No Caffeine Required**

Twitter: **@LindaMunster**

Web: **www.nocaffeinerequired.com**

ISBN 978-0-9927282-0-5

The information in this book has been compiled by way of general guidance in relation to healthy eating at work and should not be interpreted as a substitute for medical advice. It is your responsibility to determine, through obtaining appropriate medical advice, that you are fit and well and that the guidelines and services offered are suitable for you. Please consult your GP (1) if you're in any way concerned about your health, (2) you are very overweight, (3) before commencing any exercise regime (4) if you have an existing medical condition that could be affected by changing your diet (5) if you believe you have an eating disorder (6) if you are pregnant or planning a pregnancy.

We try to make sure that all information contained in this book (and provided by us to you as part of any services or products) is correct, but we do not accept any liability for any error or omission and exclude all liability for any action you may take or loss or injury you may suffer (direct or indirect including loss of pay, profit, opportunity or time, pain and suffering, any indirect, consequential or special loss, however arising) as a result of relying on any information in this book or provided through any service supplied by us to you.

Munster Books

Printed by CreateSpace

First Edition

For

Mum and Dad

Ronny, Emily and Ben

Acknowledgements

This book wouldn't have been possible without a number of people who have supported, cajoled and kept me on track over the past few months.

So in no particular order I would like to thank my editor Corinne Millar for working her magic, cartoonist Caroline Chapple for her wonderful illustrations, Rachel at Kaizen Design for the fabulous cover, Susanne Madsen for her impeccable coaching skills and Suzette Coon for her helpful advice and input.

I would also like to thank the inspirational Raymond Aaron and his team for giving me the practical and motivational tools I needed to complete this book.

I am also very grateful to Patrick Holford for agreeing to write the foreword. I have read so many of Patrick's books and am delighted he has now read mine.

Last but not least, a huge thanks to my dear clients who inspired me to write the book in the first place ... and of course my wonderful family and friends for their support and patience.

Contents

Foreword by Patrick Holford i

Preface iii

Special Bonuses iv

Health and Energy Monitor (pre-programme) v

Introduction: Desperately Seeking Energy 1

Chapter 1: The Energy Drainers 6

Chapter 2: The POWER Eating Programme™ 22

Chapter 3: POWER Meal Solutions 43

Chapter 4: Planning your POWER Meals 51

Chapter 5: Smart Ways to Execute your POWER Plan 58

Chapter 6: POWER Eating After Hours 70

Chapter 7: Boost the POWER, Bust the Stress 74

Chapter 8: Recipes 83

Conclusion: POWER Eating in a Nutshell 96

Next steps 100

Health and Energy Monitor (after 4 weeks) 102

Appendix 1: Glycemic Index & Load of Common Foods 103

Appendix 2: Resources 106

Appendix 3: Glossary 109

Foreword by Patrick Holford

A child once said in an exam howler that 'man is a knackered ape'. This is certainly an apt description of modern man. Linda Munster, in her excellent POWER Eating Programme™, gives the naked truth about why so many people are walking around tired all the time, propped up and craving sugar and caffeine to keep going.

In our research, now involving over 100,000 people, we know that the symptoms that most predict a person who will struggle with their weight are: an inability to get going in the morning without a caffeinated drink or something sweet; a craving for a dessert or sweet at the end of a meal; energy slumps in the afternoon; and feeling tired much of the time.

Unwittingly, we have become like drug addicts – with legal 'uppers' such as sugar, caffeine and nicotine to keep us going and 'downers' in the former of alcohol to relax. As nutritional therapists, we know why – but so too does the food and drink industry. They have learnt how to press our buttons and thus delightful temptations are available 'within an arm's reach of desire'.

Like a wave breaking, the burst of energy from instant sugar and caffeine leads to more tiredness and stress, followed by cravings for more stimulants and relaxants. It's a vicious cycle and if you don't break out of it things are going to get worse, not just stay the same.

However, there is another way to get energy and it's clean, with no downsides at all. In fact, the only side-effects are all good – less risk for diseases from cancer to Alzheimer's; easy weight control; less expensive; and better sleep. To convert to this cleaner fuel takes a few days and losing a few entrenched habits but, as you do so you'll find your cravings fall away. It is not difficult but it takes a few weeks to break any habit.

Modern living is out of sync with our natural design, but doesn't have to be. With so much information streaming in we need, now more than ever, to feed our brains as well as our bodies, the best fuel possible to sustain energy and health.

Linda's POWER Eating Programme™ is an intelligent person's way to put into action the principles that have emerged from thousands of studies in nutrition in the past few decades, but also echo the ancients, such as Hippocrates who said more than 2000 years ago 'When enough sins (against Nature) have accumulated, disease develops'.

Read this book, follow the POWER Eating Programme™ and feel the difference. You will not be disappointed.

Patrick Holford – founder of the Institute for Optimum Nutrition, author of the Low GL Diet Bible and Optimum Nutrition Bible

Preface

Six years ago I qualified as a nutritional therapist at the renowned Institute for Optimum Nutrition (ION) in London which was founded by leading nutritional expert, Patrick Holford. Since then I have given nutritional advice to hundreds of individuals, helping them with a range of health issues including eczema, IBS, headaches, low mood, high cholesterol, high blood pressure, arthritis and weight loss.

I also run Zest4life nutrition & weight loss courses, based on Patrick Holford's low-GL eating principles, and these have provided me with the perfect platform to share my knowledge and passion with members of the public. These programmes have helped many of my clients to not only lose a significant amount of weight, but also to regain their health and vitality and lead fuller lives.

The majority of my clients are busy working people who, over time, have developed poor eating habits and generally feel tired and under par. I never tire of hearing how a few simple dietary changes can make such a difference to how they feel, and almost without exception the first thing they notice is increased energy levels.

With this in mind, I devised my unique POWER Eating Programme™ to help improve energy levels, wellbeing and productivity at work, which could have the added benefit of fewer days taken off sick.

My POWER @ Work lunchtime seminars have been well received by a number of companies and the positive feedback from employees has convinced me of the need for this book.

I hope you will benefit from my POWER Eating Programme™ and enjoy long lasting energy throughout your busy days.

Linda Munster

The POWER Nutrition Coach

Special Bonuses

A number of special offers and bonuses are offered in this book. Please go to **www.nocaffeinerequired**.com to benefit from the following:

FREE* 5-Day Food Diary Review

Download the POWER Food & Energy diary.
Write down your food intake for 5 days then return
to info@nocaffeinerequired.com
for FREE analysis and feedback on your food choices.
* Offer limited to the first 100 applicants

POWER Meal Plans & Shopping List

Receive your free menu plans and shopping list. The
POWER Shopping List will give you a list of all the
items you need to get started.

"Recommend Us" Incentive

Take a look at our POWER @ Work services, including
lunchtime talks and half day workshops based on the
unique POWER Eating Programme™.
As a reward for introducing us to your company you
will receive a FREE half-hour private telephone /
Skype consultation plus a two-week food diary review
with one of our qualified nutrition consultants.

10% Discount from The Natural Dispensary

For your special discount on supplements and a
number of healthy snacks, register on our website
and request the 10% discount code.

Health and Energy Monitor (pre-programme)

It is really important to measure your progress, so before you start the POWER Eating Programme™ fill in the form below and add up your scores to work out your current health and energy status. Repeat the exercise after four weeks (see page 102) and celebrate your success!

How are you feeling?	Disagree................Agree				
I feel tired most of the time	1	2	3	4	5
I have poor memory / concentration	1	2	3	4	5
I am often stressed / anxious	1	2	3	4	5
I am prone to colds, flu, infections	1	2	3	4	5
I am overweight	1	2	3	4	5
I often have mood swings	1	2	3	4	5
I am prone to hormonal symptoms	1	2	3	4	5
I am prone to headaches	1	2	3	4	5
I don't sleep well	1	2	3	4	5
I suffer from indigestion / bloating	1	2	3	4	5
I am often constipated	1	2	3	4	5

Your total score: [ ]   Ideal score: 14 or less

How's your energy / blood sugar?	Disagree................Agree				
I need coffee, tea or something sweet to get me going in the morning	1	2	3	4	5
I have less energy than I used to	1	2	3	4	5
I feel tired 20 minutes after getting up	1	2	3	4	5
I often crave sweet foods, bread, chocolate, cereal, pasta	1	2	3	4	5
I often have energy slumps during the day	1	2	3	4	5
I often crave a coffee / something sweet after meals	1	2	3	4	5
I often overreact to stress	1	2	3	4	5
I find it difficult to concentrate at work	1	2	3	4	5
I often feel too tired to exercise	1	2	3	4	5
I am gaining / finding it hard to lose weight	1	2	3	4	5

Your total score: [ ]   Ideal score: 12 or less

Introduction: Desperately Seeking Energy

Picture the scene: you're woken up brusquely by your alarm clock and, still semi-comatose, you hit the snooze button and allow your head to sink back into the pillow. It takes a while before you are able to drag yourself out of bed and, making your way into the kitchen, you flick the kettle switch, impatiently waiting for your first brew of the day. Gradually, you start to feel 'normal' and ready to start your day. You never have time for breakfast and on the way to the station, grab a muffin and another shot of caffeine while you're at it.

You arrive at the office, still feeling not quite with it and the first thing you see is the much loved vending machine which tempts you to buy biscuits and yet more coffee. Suitably fuelled, you deal with your various tasks and then at lunchtime it is off to the sandwich shop where you choose a baguette with cheese washed down with a cola drink. By mid-afternoon though, your energy is fading fast and you need another pick-me-up. Once again the trusty vending machine is there to oblige. By the end of the day your head is fuzzy, your energy rock bottom and you can't wait to get home and crash on the sofa – after devouring a pizza, that is.

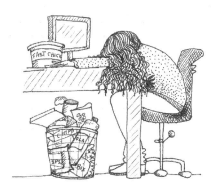

If any of this sounds familiar, then you are energetically challenged, but by no means alone. In fact, you could be forgiven for thinking this is normal behaviour given that as a nation we consume around 165 million cups of tea and 70 million cups of coffee per day (UK Tea Council). Caffeine comes in many forms and whether it's a latte, cappuccino, espresso, filtered coffee, instant coffee, cola drinks, the Great British cuppa or chocolate, we're clearly all hooked on the stuff. What's more, it's also considered perfectly normal to have a couple of biscuits with your cup of tea - remember the advert "A drink's too wet without one"?

Yet there's nothing normal about continuously pumping our bodies with caffeine and sugary snacks and the evidence is plain to see – sluggish, tired and overweight people are an all too familiar sight in the fast paced world in which we live.

Of course, there's nothing wrong with enjoying the occasional cup of tea or coffee; indeed they are a source of healthy antioxidants (see Glossary on page 109) provided they're not laden with sugar and cream. What is worrying though is the reliance on caffeine and sugar to keep you going, not least because you are neglecting the bounty of natural foods that could make you feel so much better.

So how does this sound instead? You wake up feeling ready to bounce out of bed and embrace the day. You drink some revitalising lemon in water and make a nourishing breakfast that will sustain you through the morning. Throughout the day you remain focused, mentally alert and able to deal calmly with the challenges of your work. By the time you get home, you still have energy left to enjoy your evening. Finally, after a satisfying, productive day you have a good night's sleep, ready to take on the next day with energy and zest for life.

If you find this second scenario appealing then read on.

Who this book is for

This book has been written for busy people who struggle to get through the day without resorting to endless stimulants to keep themselves awake. If you're one of these people and you're looking for more natural solutions to stay energised all day, then this book will help you do just that. Although I have written with the desk-bound office worker in mind, my book can benefit anyone who desires more energy and is prepared to make some simple changes to the way they eat and drink.

Energy at work

Making good food choices during the working day is essential to your overall health and wellbeing as most of us spend at least eight hours a day at work. Low energy levels are likely to result in reduced productivity at work – and vending machines will do you no favours.

Link between food and energy

Over the years, many of my clients have come to me complaining that they constantly feel drowsy and fuzzy-headed. As the day progresses, their energy levels flag and they wrongly assume that this is an inevitable consequence of the ageing process. It doesn't occur to them that it might be down to the food they eat, as they truly believe they have a 'balanced' diet. However, once they start to make some simple nutritional changes and to consume the right fuel, it takes very little time before they regain their energy and vitality. As clichéd as it might sound, we most definitely are what we eat!

Case study:

Take Deb – a 48 year old teacher who came to me with energy levels on the floor and was frequently taking time off work due to ill health. After following my healthy eating plan for a few weeks, Deb noticed a dramatic change in her energy levels and was delighted to no longer have to go to bed at 9pm. She emailed me one day to say that for the first time in her 20-year career she hadn't once phoned in sick over the winter term. The secret? A few simple changes to her eating habits – a true testimony to the power of food.

Indeed, I was exactly like Deb myself back in the days when I didn't know much about nutrition. Working in a pressurised corporate world with deadlines, demanding management and long hours, I frequently found myself dozing off in front of the computer in the early afternoon after a giant baguette. It didn't feel good at all and what's more, my productivity levels suffered so my employer definitely wasn't getting the best from me.

Now I can't blame anyone for their confusion because all around us we are assailed by conflicting messages about what to eat. Literally every week we are faced with a different diet or product that promises to change our lives for good. I'm not suggesting that these are all wrong but my feeling is if we could just stick to natural, unadulterated foods and cut down on the processed, refined products, then we can't go far wrong.

Energy plus ...

Having more energy means you are able to concentrate better, achieve more and enjoy a highly productive day without crashing out half way through it. Other benefits include better mood, a greater ability to deal with stress, improved quality of sleep and even weight loss – a very welcome bonus indeed!

You will also find that you'll have more energy to enjoy life outside the workplace. For example, not only does Deb feel better and more energised but she has used her newfound energy to run the 5k Race for Life and to climb Mount Snowdon – all beyond her wildest dreams before she changed her diet. So the benefits of energy can be truly life-changing and I wish to make it as easy as possible for you to regain the energy that is rightfully yours.

Coming up ...

The purpose of this book is not only to share my knowledge with you, but also to help you put it into practice. That is why I devised the POWER Eating Programme™ so that you'll know exactly what to eat – and what not to eat – and how to go about making a plan that works for you.

Thus in the following chapters you will first learn about the foods and drinks that hinder your natural energy supply, causing you to struggle to get through the day. You'll then discover the delicious, nutritious foods that will help fuel your body and mind, keeping you focused and productive all day long.

I shall then help you plan and prepare your foods and get you started on making some small changes which I know can make a big difference to your wellbeing.

There will also be ideas on how you can maximise the benefits of this new way of eating by incorporating exercise and even chill time into your busy day.

Of course, whilst this book focuses on meal solutions for your working day, you need to apply the principles to every meal. So I discuss ways of keeping the energy going after hours too so you can live a healthier life – and all without the need for stimulants.

Finally, no book on food would be complete without recipes so I've gathered together some of my favourites and you'll see they're really very simple and practical.

Once you have read this book you will always know what to choose for optimal health, energy and vitality and my hope for you is that you'll never wish to turn back.

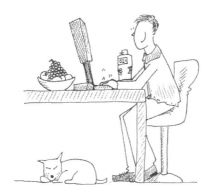

Chapter 1: The Energy Drainers

It's simple: if we have an abundance of energy we feel positive, motivated and more able to achieve. If we are low in energy, we feel incapable, unenthusiastic and unproductive.

In this chapter, we will look at the science behind how the body makes energy from food and why relying on endless stimulants such as caffeine, sugar and alcohol is undermining your energy levels and your long term health.

What is energy?

Energy is essential to life and defined as "the strength and vitality required for sustained physical or mental activity". The basic law of energy is that while it is everywhere, it can never be created or destroyed but simply transformed from one state to another. Thus the energy in what we eat and drink is ultimately converted into fuel that the body can use, known as adenosine triphosphate (ATP) and this powers everything we do. The complex series of chemical reactions that convert food into energy is your metabolism which never stops working; even when you are at rest you still need energy for 'hidden' functions such as breathing, circulation, digestion, growth and repair.

Not all calories are created equal!

Although all foods give us energy, that doesn't mean all foods enhance our energy in the same way. Energy from food is commonly measured in calories and conventional wisdom is that a calorie is a calorie, so eating 100 calories of white bread would give you the same kind of energy as 100 calories of broccoli.

However, not all calories are created equal, and there are other important factors which affect energy such as the nutrient content of food. An efficient metabolism requires vital nutrients such as B-complex vitamins and Omega 3 fatty acids to help our bodies convert food into energy, so it is important to eat *nutrient-dense* foods such as vegetables, fruit and nuts. *Energy-dense* foods such as white bread and pasta are high in calories but low or deficient in nutrients, so it stands to reason that these foods will not generate energy efficiently. So instead of counting calories, there is a far more accurate way to determine the energy potential of our food and that is to look at the effect it has on your blood sugar.

Blood sugar and energy

During the process of digestion, *all carbohydrates* – whether in bread, grains, cereals, pasta, sweets, juices, fruits and vegetables – end up as the simple sugar glucose which is the preferred fuel for our body, including the brain. Glucose is then absorbed into the bloodstream as blood sugar. In response to the rise in blood sugar, the hormone insulin is released from the pancreas and escorts the glucose to your cells which then convert it into energy in their specialised 'powerhouses', the mitochondria. Your blood sugar levels correlate directly with your energy levels so if your blood sugar is low, your energy will be low too - hence the feeling of fatigue.

Dietary fat can also be broken down for energy and, in the absence of carbs and fat, protein can be used. So the body is always able to manufacture energy from whatever we eat.

This may sound simple but different foods (especially carbs) affect your blood sugar, and therefore your energy levels, in very different ways. So let us take a look at the types of food and drink that throw a spanner in the energy works.

The Blood Sugar Rollercoaster

Carbohydrate foods are categorised as either *simple*, containing refined sugars, or *complex*, composed of starches, fibre, vitamins and minerals (see next chapter for more on complex carbs).

Simple carbohydrate foods are often regarded as the 'bad' carbs as they include refined white flour products such as white bread and pasta, and sugary foods such as biscuits and soft drinks. Lacking in nutrients and fibre, these energy-dense, fast-release foods provide no material for the body to break down, so they enter the bloodstream at lightning speed, causing a rapid surge in blood sugar and insulin levels. This gives you a short energy boost, but the sugar is used up all too quickly by the cells. Before long your blood sugar/energy levels plummet, potentially leaving you tired, irritable and unable to concentrate. What's more, you end up craving more sugary carbs as this is your body's way to get your energy up again. So you continue on this energy rollercoaster all day, every day, feeling increasingly worn out and making poor, unhealthy food choices on the way.

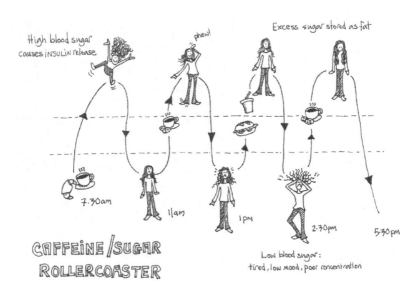

High blood sugar causes INSULIN release

phew!

Excess sugar stored as fat

7.30am

11am

1PM

2.30pm

5.30pm

CAFFEINE/SUGAR ROLLERCOASTER

Low blood sugar: tired, low mood, poor concentration

Stress and sugar

Eating this way causes a state of stress in the body, a huge energy drainer if ever there was one. This is because whenever your blood sugar plummets, another hormone kicks in to release sugar into the bloodstream, restoring blood sugar and energy levels, albeit temporarily. That hormone is adrenaline (also known as epinephrine), the 'fight or flight' stress hormone secreted by the adrenal glands with the evolutionary purpose of dealing with an 'emergency'. Adrenaline is great as a backup energy supply because it enables us to keep going and get the job done, but we must not rely on it as it can seriously affect our health ...

In fact, according to BUPA (2011) nearly half a million people are taking time off work each year due to work-related stress which they believe is making them ill.

Stress in today's world is very different to that faced by our primitive ancestors but the body's response is just the same – our heart beats faster, our blood pressure rises as the body can't tell the difference between the threat of a sabre-tooth tiger or a tax bill! However, rather than use up the adrenaline-fuelled energy for fleeing or fighting the wild beast and allowing the body to return to normal, we seethe at our desk allowing the stress to build up – rather like a pressure cooker with no outlet to let off steam. This constant state of stress can eventually tax your adrenals (see Glossary on page 109) and lead to burnout.

So not only do we feel stressed by external pressures of modern life, but we add to the problem by eating sugary foods which create even more stress in the body – as if you weren't stressed enough already!

Furthermore, any excess sugar the body cannot use is stored in the body as **fat** so not only do you feel increasingly tired and depleted as the day wears on, but you gain weight too.

Thus, the effect of sugary, refined foods is clear – it wears you out, causes stress in the body, can make you sluggish and overweight. Hardly a recipe for an energy-filled day!

To make matters worse, regular consumption of these highly processed, sugary foods will also increase your risk of developing cardiovascular disease and type-2 diabetes, so avoid the following as much as possible.

⊘   White bread, white pasta, white rice, cakes, biscuits, muffins, flapjacks, confectionery, sugary breakfast cereals, cereal bars, fizzy drinks, juices and squashes.

However, avoiding sugar is sometimes easier said than done, partly because it can be so difficult to spot and also because it's so addictive. Rest assured though that once you start to reduce your sugar intake, its addictiveness starts to wear off - so let me help you be sugar savvy.

The sugar menace

Sugar is everywhere, ranging from the obvious places like sweets, biscuits, cakes and chocolate but also sneakily hidden inside flavoured low-fat or fat-free products. For example, to compensate for the missing fat, manufacturers add sugar to low-fat fruit yoghurts, making them more palatable. Then there are breakfast cereals, muesli bars, granola and flapjacks – as healthy as they sound they are all heavily laced with sugar.

Get food label savvy - the many guises of sugar

Even if the word 'sugar' doesn't appear on the label it could well be lurking in there somewhere. Sugar appears under many other names such as syrup, evaporated cane juice, concentrated fruit juice, molasses, honey and maltodextrin. Brown sugar is no better than white as demerara, muscovado, cane sugar still have very few, if any nutrients, and will disrupt your blood sugar just the same.

Look out too for anything ending in '–ose' e.g. maltose, dextrose, glucose, sucrose (table sugar), fructose, high fructose corn syrup (USA), glucose-fructose syrup (Europe). These are all sugars in disguise and at best, they will only provide a short-term energy boost, leaving you tired in no time at all.

How can I check how much sugar is in a food?

The first sign is where sugar appears in the ingredients list – if it's near the top, it's one of the dominant ingredients and should be avoided. The nutritional panel on the food label will display carbohydrates 'of which sugars', and this tells you just how much sugar is in your product. The following table shows you the sugar content of some common foods and drinks.

Product	Amount of sugar (g)
150 g pot low-fat flavoured yoghurt	26
330 ml/12 oz can Coca Cola Classic	39
330 ml / 12 oz Fanta	32
50g Jordan's Natural Muesli	12
Kellogg's Nutrigrain Cereal Bar	11
Starbucks low-fat blueberry muffin	57
30g bowl of Cornflakes + s/skimmed milk	9
2 digestive biscuits	5
KitKat (2-finger bar)	10

Source: www.myfitnesspal.com

Put into context, four grams of sugar are equivalent to approximately one teaspoon so you could be eating over six teaspoons of sugar in a single pot of low-fat flavoured (e.g. vanilla, raspberry) yoghurt, nine cubes of sugar in a can of coke and fourteen teaspoons in a muffin!

What's considered an acceptable amount of sugar?

Guidelines set by the Food Standards Agency (FSA) state that 15g of sugars or more per 100g is high and you can see from the table how many foods contain a lot more than this. 5g or less per 100g is low so in order to cure yourself of that sweet tooth you need to be aiming as low as possible.

Save sugar, save energy. Just think, if you switched your low-fat, flavoured yoghurt for a natural unsweetened one, you could be saving approximately five teaspoons of sugar a day, 35 per week, 140 per month and a whopping 1,680 per year! You'd be saving energy as your body wouldn't have to use up its valuable resources trying to process all that surplus sugar.

Don't believe everything you read on the label!

Despite the extensive lists of vitamins and minerals that you see on your cereal box, you need to know that these have not occurred naturally in the cereal. This is because the germ and the bran, the most nutritious parts of the original whole grain, are removed during the refining process, leaving the rather unsatisfying endosperm which contains only small amounts of vitamins and minerals. The nutrients in your cereal are just added back in a form that's difficult to absorb, together with plenty of energy-sapping sugar, so the body derives little benefit from them.

Whilst fibre is an essential component of the diet, I'm not a great fan of the fibre that's added back into cereals as it comes from wheat bran and can be harsh on a sensitive gut. Bran is also high in phytates which can actually inhibit the absorption of minerals such as calcium and iron, essential for energy production. There are many other sources of fibre which occur naturally and you will find out about these in the next chapter.

Neither should you be impressed by a long list of strange sounding ingredients as many of them will be preservatives and additives which contribute nothing to your energy and wellbeing – in fact, if you can't pronounce them put the product straight back on the shelf! The fewer ingredients the better as the closer to nature the product is the more wholesome and healthy it is likely to be.

Thus, the loss of vital nutrients together with the addition of sugar creates a double whammy on our energy levels. Yet vast quantities of these 'empty' foods are enjoyed by millions every minute of the day, and that's because sugar is so irresistible.

Why is sugar so addictive?

I've lost count of the number of clients who come to me with sugar cravings and are horrified when they realise they may have to give it up. This is because sugar is highly addictive and many anti-sugar campaigners liken it to controlled drugs. Amongst them is Dr. Robert Lustig, a leading US obesity expert whose book "Fat Chance: The Bitter Sweet Truth" has been recently published. Lustig believes sugar is an addictive toxin and should be regulated in the same way as cigarettes. "We need to wean ourselves off. We need to de-sweeten our lives. We need to make sugar a treat, not a diet staple," he says, and I couldn't agree more.

The reason for sugar's addictiveness is that it has no nutritional value so it can never actually satisfy the real needs of the body. It also temporarily boosts the 'feel good' hormone serotonin but because the effect is so short-lived you end up craving more and more. Furthermore, sugar, in particular fructose (which forms the sweeter half of sucrose, the other half being glucose), doesn't send a signal to the brain that you are full, so there's no mechanism known to the body that makes you stop eating the stuff. You can therefore become addicted, overweight, permanently hungry and tired.

You may be concerned that you will find it difficult to give up this sweet substance but please don't worry – if you follow the advice in this book and give your body what it needs your cravings will reduce in no time.

Other perils of sugar

Sugar is also associated with a host of other health problems and risks:

- Weakens your immune system so can make you sick

- Can cause premature ageing and wrinkles

- Increases the risk of diabetes

- Can damage the artery walls leading to raised cholesterol and heart disease

- Associated with hyperactivity

- Can encourage yeast overgrowth (candida)

- Can cause fatigue

- Can make you anxious and irritable

- Can cause gum disease and tooth decay

What about artificial sweeteners?

Aspartame (NutraSweet), sucralose (Splenda) and saccharin can all be found in so-called 'diet' foods and drinks. As they contain zero calories, they are assumed to be good for us. However, in my opinion anything artificial needs to be regarded with suspicion and reported side-effects of aspartame include headaches, fatigue, depression, joint pain and nausea. Ironically, artificial sweeteners also stimulate appetite so despite the lack of calories they can actually make you hungry. Please refer to page 37 for more on the natural sweeteners I do recommend.

The less obvious sources of sugar: fruit and starchy vegetables

Ever eaten an apple and felt hungry shortly afterwards? Potatoes, dates, pineapple, mango, grapes, bananas and even carrots can also upset blood sugar balance if eaten in excess, despite containing natural sugars and nutrients galore. As far as the body is concerned, sugar is sugar regardless of its source, and too much of it will cause a spike in blood sugar followed by a fall. As these natural foods don't come with a nutrition label, we need to refer to the 'Richter Scale of Foods', the glycemic index or glycemic load to find out how they affect our blood sugar and therefore our energy levels.

The glycemic index and glycemic load

The glycemic index (GI) measures how different carbohydrates affect your blood sugar after they are eaten and digested. Based on scores between 1 and 100 (100 being the equivalent of glucose) anything above 70 is considered high-GI, as these foods will cause a rapid rise in your blood sugar, followed by the inevitable crash. Foods rated below 50 are low-GI and will generally have a much more favourable impact on your blood sugar, giving you longer lasting energy.

The glycemic index, however, can sometimes be confusing as watermelon, for example, has a high GI score of 72 which is enough to put you off eating it. In fact you would need to devour the entire watermelon for your blood sugar to rise that high, but the GI score doesn't take quantity into account.

The glycemic load (GL), on the other hand, takes GI a step further as it tells you exactly **how much** carbohydrate you need to eat to keep your blood sugar balanced and your energy levels stable. Furthermore, whilst GI scores only apply to single foods, GL can determine the effect of a whole meal on your blood sugar. The presence of protein and fats, for example, can slow down the release of sugar into your bloodstream, sustaining your energy levels for longer. Thus, a whole plate of pasta with a tomato sauce is high GL as it is primarily carbohydrate and will not satisfy you for long, whereas a handful of pasta with a piece of chicken and vegetables will have a much lower GL and therefore sustain you for longer.

For one serving of food, a GL over 20 is considered high, 11-19 is medium and below 10 is low. In the case of the watermelon, one slice would only be 4 GLs as it contains only a small amount of sugar and the rest is mostly water. The GL method, therefore, is a more accurate indicator of how much a meal is likely to affect your blood sugar / energy levels. This is the essence of my POWER Eating Programme™ which you will read about in the following chapters.

As a rule of thumb though, high-GI or high-GL foods such as the refined, processed foods already discussed, need to be avoided as they will only provide short-term energy whilst low-GI/GL should be your foods of choice and will be discussed in detail in the next chapter. See Appendix 1 on page 103 for the glycemic index and glycemic load of common foods or for a more complete list go to **www.glycemicindex.com**.

In short, for sustained energy you need to avoid overloading your body with sugar, whether it comes as a sweetener in your products or in the form of refined carbohydrates that turn very quickly into sugar, including too much sweet fruit.

Caffeine

As already noted, caffeinated drinks are hugely popular and a whopping 120,000 tonnes of caffeine is consumed per annum on our planet.

How does it work and why do we like it so much?

Caffeine is the go-to energy booster. It is a stimulant which according to The Journal of Neuroscience is the "most consumed psychoactive drug in the world". Caffeine works by blocking the brain chemical, adenosine that slows us down and makes us sleep, so instead of dropping off in front of the computer, we wake up and get the job done – keeping the boss happy in the process. It also raises levels of the 'feel good' chemicals dopamine and serotonin, elevating our mood and keeping us alert. So it's no wonder we get hooked on the stuff: it makes us feel happier, more energised and productive – all within a few minutes.

How much caffeine should we consume?

The maximum daily limit for caffeine recommended by the UK Food Standards Agency is 400mg which is equivalent to four or five cups of coffee a day and the table below shows the main sources and caffeine content of the world's favourite drug.

Approximate caffeine content of popular drinks and food

Beverage / food	Caffeine (mg)	Quantity
Instant Coffee	100	Average mug
Filter coffee	150	Average mug
Black tea	75	Average mug
Coca-Cola	32	1 can
Pepsi	37.5	1 can
Red Bull	114	355 ml can
Plain dark chocolate	50	50g bar

Plain milk chocolate	25	50g bar
Starbucks Coffee Grande	330	16 fl oz /460 ml mug
Green tea *	25	8 fl oz / 230 ml cup
White tea *	15	8 fl oz / 230 ml cup

Source: Bournemouth University (www.buzz.bournemouth.ac.uk March 2013)

* Green and white tea contain less caffeine than black tea and higher amounts of the amino acid theanine which has a calming effect, taking the edge off the caffeine. See chapter 2 for more on the benefits of these teas.

It doesn't take much to reach 400 mg and for serial caffeine drinkers on 8-10 coffees a day, they have exceeded their limit in no time. Of course, many energy drinks contain both caffeine and sugar, providing a double hit on your energy levels.

In my opinion, and judging by the effect it has on my clients, even 400 mg is far too much caffeine to stay naturally energised and healthy. Indeed, only 200 mg is recommended during pregnancy as it may induce miscarriage - a strong indicator that this drug is not as life enhancing as we would like to think.

What's wrong with caffeine?

Caffeine is addictive. Having the occasional cup to get through a particular work assignment is fine but frequent use can have harmful effects. This is because the brain gets used to caffeine, so rather than just enjoying the occasional boost, you end up needing more and more to keep your energy levels up. If you can't get your fix, your serotonin levels drop resulting in feelings of tiredness, irritability and poor concentration, so back you go again on that adrenaline-fuelled energy rollercoaster – you're hooked and can no longer do without it.

Interestingly, research at Bristol University (2010) showed that caffeine doesn't actually make us any more alert at all - it's simply compensating for the fatiguing effects of caffeine withdrawal, making us feel 'normal' again when we consume it.

Caffeine upsets your blood sugar. We've already seen the adrenaline-sugar connection and caffeine also stimulates adrenaline to release sugar into the bloodstream to give you that instant energy boost. So whether you add sugar to your coffee or not, caffeine can upset your blood sugar balance.

Caffeine stresses you out. As a stimulant, caffeine is putting your body in a state of prolonged stress, as if you didn't have enough stress in your life! This permanent adrenaline rush pushes you to the limits and makes you think you're capable of doing more than your body can actually handle. So you carry on working, achieving, taking on the world until you eventually burn out and the wheels grind to a sudden halt.

Frequent caffeine consumption can lead to *poor eating habits* as caffeinated beverages are often paired with something sweet like a biscuit, a muffin or a flapjack, all readily available in our fashionable coffee shops. In other words, it often comes with a dose of sugar and fat to supposedly keep you satisfied, denying you the opportunity to eat something nourishing and sustaining.

Caffeine is a *diuretic* which means it's dehydrating, making the fluids in your body less able to deliver nutrients to different parts of the body.

Last but not least, caffeine can *disturb your sleep.* As caffeine can stay in your system for up to twelve hours, its effects continue long after your latte has been consumed. A good night's sleep is essential for a productive day, so if caffeine is disturbing your sleep you're bound to feel fuzzy headed the following day.

So whilst tea and coffee can be enjoyable drinks and the occasional cup won't do you any harm, it's the serial caffeine drinkers that I worry about as their dependence on this drug is likely to have adverse effects on their health. In the short term, it can make you anxious, irritable, stressed and jittery and cause headaches and heart palpitations. In the long term, the body can come down with an almighty crash leading to chronic fatigue (ME), raised blood pressure, depression, insomnia and heart disease. Ultimately it can sap all your natural energy and burn you out.

But I need my cup of coffee to get me going in the morning ...

Do you? I've come across many caffeine junkies who are concerned about giving up their trusty morning cup of tea or coffee but when they follow the advice from this book and start the day with something more revitalising and natural, such as a mug of warm lemon water, or just good old-fashioned water, their head feels clearer, they have a steadier supply of energy and they feel so much better.

So no, you don't need your coffee any more than you need that sweet biscuit to get your energy levels up half-way through the morning. My goal is to show you what your body actually does need in order to stay energised throughout the day and to challenge the belief that you must have caffeine to keep you going.

Top tip for reducing caffeine consumption

Don't go cold turkey unless you're prepared to endure a mighty caffeine withdrawal headache for the next couple of days. Just gradually reduce your intake of caffeine over several days to acclimatise your body to the new regime.

In short, sugar, refined carbs and caffeine can all play havoc with your blood sugar, giving you the peaks and troughs that are wearing you out.

Other Energy Drainers

Fatty foods and heavy meals

Chips, burgers and pizzas are all very hard to digest. To aid digestion, blood is diverted from the brain to your digestive organs and this can take up to eight hours. So with your energy directed towards your stomach you're bound to feel far less energetic.

Skipping meals

Skipping meals, especially breakfast when you haven't eaten for several hours, can also lead to low blood sugar levels, and therefore low energy. If you never feel hungry first thing, it's probably because you've had a caffeine fix which made the adrenaline pump sugar into your bloodstream and we've already seen the effect of adrenaline on our systems.

Don't believe for a minute that if you eat less, you'll lose weight – in fact, quite the opposite is true as Lorraine discovered when she followed the POWER Eating Programme™.

Case study:

Lorraine had been feeling out of sorts for a while – low energy, low mood, weight gain. She came to my POWER Eating seminar one evening at her office hoping to find a solution and couldn't believe that her problem was quite simple: she wasn't eating enough. She generally skipped breakfast and she would eat lots of fruit during the day with fruit yoghurt and then a reasonable evening meal but her body had basically shut down. So she started the POWER programme and after just 4 weeks she'd lost 11 lbs and felt great. She sent me her food diary* every week which I analysed for her and this helped her to stay motivated and on track.

* Don't forget that you too can register for your FREE 5-day food diary analysis – see page **Error! Bookmark not defined.** for details of this and other bonuses.

If you don't eat enough, your body will make the very wise decision of going into 'starvation mode' whereby it holds on to your fat for the perceived lean times ahead. Instead of fat, it lets you have some muscle for energy, but losing muscle cuts your metabolic rate and makes it very difficult to drop the pounds.

Alcohol

Considered both a stimulant and a depressant, alcohol can have a disruptive effect on your blood sugar levels especially as it goes straight to the bloodstream. It also places an unnecessary burden on your liver which has to work harder to detoxify it, thus leaving less energy for you to do other things. So alcohol during the day is definitely not recommended.

Cigarettes

The adverse effects of smoking are well known and tobacco is also a major contributor to the blood sugar / energy rollercoaster. This is because, like caffeine, it stimulates adrenaline to release sugar into the bloodstream giving you the short term high, which is shortly followed by a drop in mood and before long you become addicted. Smoking also depletes the body of nutrients such as vitamin C, so your energy and immunity are both compromised.

In summary, if you wish to last all day without crashing half way through, you will need to avoid these energy draining foods, drinks and stimulants as much as possible and to eat light meals that are easy to digest.

In the next chapter I will reveal my POWER Eating Programme™ that will help you regain your energy and vitality and give you a smoother ride throughout your day.

Chapter 2: The POWER Eating Programme™

Now you know what drains your energy, let's focus on how you can boost your working day. To help you make the right food choices, my unique POWER Eating Programme™ is based on an acronym representing the five essential components of every meal:

P   Protein

O   Oils and Fats

W Whole Grains and Starchy Vegetables

E   Energising Vegetables and Fruit

R   Revitalising drinks

And that's it, just five powerful letters that can keep you energised, focused and productive throughout your busy day.

The POWER plate

The plate shows you the 'balance of POWER' you need to achieve in order to derive maximum energy from your meals. Each component of the plate is discussed on the following pages.

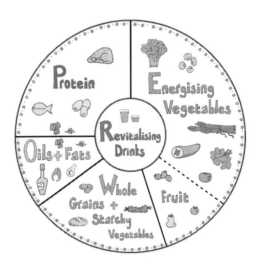

| P | O | W | E | R | **Protein** |

"Where's the protein?" is a question that will resonate with many of my clients. When they first show me their food diaries, 9 times out of 10 I comment on the lack of protein in their diet which usually accounts for their hunger, tiredness and lack of energy. This is because protein keeps your blood sugar balanced as it slows down the release of sugar into your bloodstream, so you stay fuller for longer, have more sustained energy and eat less - a major benefit for your waistline!

A few more facts about protein

Protein actually makes up part of all the cells and tissues in your body, including hair, skin and nails and is required for growth and repair. The body also needs protein to make enzymes that turn food into energy, hormones such as adrenaline and insulin, and neurotransmitters connected with good mood, motivation and concentration.

Protein is made up of 20 building blocks called amino acids; eight of these are essential as the body cannot make them itself, so they must come from the diet. When carbohydrate and fat is not available, the body can convert amino acids into glucose which is then used for energy.

How much protein?

I recommend that protein constitute approximately a quarter of each main meal to keep you satisfied and energised. As a rough guide this equates to the size of the palm of your hand.

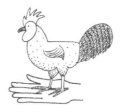

Animal sources of protein

- Meat and poultry: chicken, turkey, duck (free range, organic if possible), beef, lamb, pork (lean ham and bacon), venison, liver

- Fish and shellfish: salmon, tuna, sardines, mackerel, trout, cod, haddock, hake, sea bass, anchovies, prawns, crab, mussels

- Dairy produce: milk & yoghurt (from cow, goat or sheep); cheese eg. feta, halloumi, goat's cheese, Cheddar, Edam, parmesan, cottage cheese, cream cheese; whey protein powder

- Eggs: free range, organic if possible

Vegetable sources of protein

- Beans and pulses: aduki, kidney, butterbean, haricot (baked beans), cannellini, pinto, chickpeas, chickpeas (hummus), soya beans and products (tofu and miso), lentils

- Nuts: walnuts, macadamias, almonds, hazelnuts, Brazils, pecans, cashews, pistachios, raw peanuts, nut butters: e.g. peanut, almond or hazelnut

- Seeds: sunflower, pumpkin, sesame, chia seeds, flaxseeds (linseeds), hemp seeds, pine nuts, quinoa (technically a seed so contains protein as well as carbohydrate), tahini (sesame paste), pesto (pine nuts)

- Pea or hemp protein powders

Animal sources of protein provide the full range of amino acids and are known as complete proteins. Plant foods, on the other hand, frequently lack one or more of the essential amino acids, so if you are vegetarian you need to eat a combination of beans, pulses, vegetables and grains to ensure you are obtaining the full complement. Thus rice and lentils or baked beans on toast will provide complete protein meals.

The wonder of eggs

Eggs are a great source of protein and provide vitamins A, D, E and the B vitamins as well as many minerals including iron, magnesium, calcium and zinc. They also contain essential fatty acids. Whilst the yolk contains cholesterol, studies show no significant correlation between dietary cholesterol and blood cholesterol[1] and the lecithin in egg yolk actually assists the breakdown of cholesterol in the body. Thus, the advice to limit eggs to twice a week is totally outdated and misguided and, unless instructed otherwise by your health professional, you can happily enjoy eight eggs per week. Ideally choose organic eggs from pasture-raised 'happy' hens that have been fed on omega 3-rich flax.

Ways with eggs

Scrambled, hardboiled, soft boiled, poached, omelette, frittata, tortilla

Yoghurt

Plain, natural yoghurt is a good source of protein and contains beneficial bacteria which are vital for good digestion and immunity. These bacteria also manufacture B vitamins in the gut so play an important role in energy production.

Top tip

Include protein with every meal including snacks, so eating a few almonds with your apple, or topping your oatcake with hummus or nut butter will keep your energy going throughout the day.

---

[1] BMJ Egg Consumption and Risk of Coronary Heart Disease and Stroke: Dose-Response Meta-Analysis of Prospective Cohort Studies. Rong et al BMJ 2013

P O W E R Oils & Fats

Don't be fat phobic! Despite the demonisation of fats, most fats are actually good for you and a great source of energising fuel. The brain is made up of around 60% fat so adequate healthy fat in the diet is essential for optimal brain function and will keep your mind alert throughout the day. Like protein, fats are more satiating than carbs so keep you fuller for longer. Fat is also needed to absorb the fat-soluble vitamins A, D, E and K which are all critical to health and wellbeing.

Furthermore, the essential fatty acids, particularly Omega 3, can actually help you lose weight as they increase your metabolic rate and your ability to burn fat[2].

How much fat?

You can see from the POWER plate that around 10% of your diet needs to contain 'good' fats but because of 'fat phobia' many people fall very short of this fat quota or they eat the wrong 'bad' fats.

The 'good' fats

There are different types of healthy 'good' fats depending on their molecular structure but the following are all beneficial to our health:

Saturated fats

• Meat, poultry, butter, eggs, coconut and palm oils

These form a vital part of every cell membrane in your body, together with essential fatty acids and cholesterol, and are the preferred fuel for the heart. Contrary to popular belief these fats are good for you and many studies have shown no association between them and heart disease. As this discussion is beyond the scope of this book, please refer to Drs Mercola and Briffa in

---

[2] www.udoerasmus.com/articles/udo/from_fat_to_fit.htm

the Resources section on page 106 to learn more about the unfortunate fallacy that has been propagated for nearly 40 years that saturated fat is bad for you.

Coconut energy

I admit it: I am a total coconut addict! It has a high burning point so doesn't get damaged when heated and I use coconut oil liberally in my stir-fries, scrambled eggs, curries and even porridge! The fat in coconut is known as a medium chained triglyceride and rather than getting stored in the body as fat, it travels directly to the liver where it is converted into energy. Whilst research is in its prime, there is much evidence to suggest that coconut protects the brain and may help reverse or halt the progression of dementia (www.coconutoil.com).

Monounsaturated fats

- Avocados, olives and their oils

Staples of the 'Mediterranean' diet, these fats and their oils are essential for heart health, glowing skin and again provide an important source of energy. Studies show that olive oil keeps the heart young which can only be good news for energy and vitality.

Polyunsaturated fats

These include Omegas 3 and 6, the essential fatty acids that the body cannot manufacture itself, hence *essential*.

- Omega 3 sources: salmon, mackerel, trout, sardines, fresh tuna (not canned), flaxseeds, flax oil, chia seeds, walnuts, pasture-raised eggs.

- Omega 6 sources: most nuts and seeds such as hazelnuts, almonds, sunflower, pumpkin and sesame seeds.

Top tips

Soaking nuts in the fridge overnight makes them more digestible

Bake nuts e.g. almonds in oven on low temperature (around 150ºC, 300ºF, Gas mark 2) for half an hour until crisp and crunchy

Avoid the 'bad' fats

Whilst the above fats are essential for good health, there are some harmful fats that need to be avoided. The most dangerous are artificial trans fats, also known as hydrogenated oils, which are cheap vegetable oils that have had their molecular structure altered to become more solid, such as margarine. Note that if a fat is liquid in its natural state, then it is an oil, and that's how we should consume it. However, hydrogenation converts healthy oils into artificially saturated fats and the only advantage is an increased shelf life which should instantly arouse suspicion.

What's more, these artificial fats compete against your energising essential fats, placing a drain on your health and vitality.

🚫 Steer clear of deep-fried fast foods, margarine, crisps, shop-bought biscuits, cakes and baked goods.

These bad fats increase the risk of heart attacks, heart disease and strokes, plus they contribute to increased inflammation, diabetes and other health problems. So yes, there are some fats that you do need to be phobic about.

Cooking oils and fats

Polyunsaturated fats such as sunflower, soybean or corn oils are far less stable than saturated and monounsaturated fats and can oxidise – or 'go rancid' – if exposed to heat, light and air. Thus if these oils are used for cooking they produce large amounts of damaging free radicals (see Glossary on page 109) that can wreak havoc in our bodies. So avoid frying in sunflower oil, for example, as it turns into a **bad fat** that is harmful to our body (Erasmus, 1993. See Resources on page 109).

• Best cooking oils and fats: butter, coconut oil, ghee or olive oil.

- Best fat-based spreads: hummus (with olive oil), coconut butter (when solid), mashed avocado, tahini (sesame paste), nut butters (e.g. almond, hazelnut), butter, fish pâtés (mackerel, salmon).

- Best oils to use in dressings: extra virgin olive oil, flax (linseed) oil, sesame oil (see recipes on page 92).

🚫 Worst fat-based spread: margarine.

P O W E R Whole Grains & Starchy Veg

This is the carbohydrate-rich section of the plate where portion control is really important to keep your blood sugar balanced. You'll see that whole grains and starchy vegetables share the same space on the plate and should constitute around a **quarter** of your meal as they can all drain you if eaten in excess. However, if they are consumed in the right amounts, with other POWER components, they provide a good source of energy.

Whole grains

We've already seen that eating simple refined grains upsets our blood sugar balance resulting in an energy rollercoaster ride throughout the day. So to enjoy a smoother ride, your fuel of choice should come from complex, unrefined, low GI/GL carbohydrates.

Due to their *fibre* content, these complex whole grains take longer to digest and so release their energy slowly, leading to more stable energy levels. In addition, they provide many important vitamins, minerals and plant chemicals that keep your body well-nourished and energised. For example, B vitamins are concentrated in the bran of the grains and are an essential part of the energy production process (see POWER nutrients on page 37).

Whole grain sources

- Healthy whole grains include wholegrain bread and cereals, pumpernickel bread, rye bread, brown rice, wholemeal pasta, bulgur (cracked) wheat, barley, brown basmati rice, rolled jumbo (porridge) oats, spelt, quinoa, giant couscous, millet, soba (buckwheat) noodles.

- Best breads: wholegrain, stoneground or wholemeal bread, wholemeal wraps and pitta bread, corn wrap (gluten free), pumpernickel, rye bread, spelt bread, sourdough, soda bread, sprouted bread.

- Best crackers: oatcakes, Dr Karg spelt crackers, seeded Ryvita.

- Best breakfast cereals: oat-based muesli, granola, porridge. Second best: Weetabix, Oatibix, Shredded Wheat.

- Avoid white bread, panini, baguettes, bagels, granary, multigrain - often white bread in disguise with a few seeds and grains thrown in!

Whole grain portions

Despite their fibre and nutrients, even the 'good carbs' should not make up more than a quarter of your meal as an excess of these complex grains can still make you tired. This applies particularly to bread which is why a huge sandwich at lunch time can tire you out for the afternoon.

Using the glycemic load as discussed on page 15, these are the approximate whole grain portions you should aim to have on your plate. Following these guidelines will ensure you don't end up with too much sugar in your system which needs to be rushed out of the blood, causing an energy slump.

- 1 slice of bread
- 3 oatcakes
- 30g pasta

- 40g brown rice

- A large bowl of porridge oats

- 2 handfuls of quinoa

- 1 handful of couscous

Avoid eating these foods on their own as they need to be combined with the other sections of the plate to provide sustaining nourishment.

Moreover, controlling your carb portions will not only keep you energised, but slim too as there won't be any surplus sugar to get stored as fat. So it's a win-win situation!

Starchy vegetables

Starchy vegetables such as potatoes occupy the same section of the POWER plate as whole grains because the starches they contain are broken down into sugar at varying rates and thus have a significant effect on your blood sugar, and therefore energy levels. So you need to be mindful of how much starch is in your meals. Take a look at the starchy vegetables and the amounts recommended per meal to keep you alert and focused rather than making you drowsy. Some may surprise you ...

- 3 new potatoes or half a jacket potato

- ½ large sweet potato

- 1 large carrot

- 1 parsnip

- Half a corn on cob

- Large serving spoon of butternut squash

- 1½ tablespoons broad beans

- 1 medium beetroot

- 50g peas

So if your lunch consists of a giant jacket potato with some sweetcorn and grated carrot and maybe a slice of bread on the side, it's hardly surprising you feel tired! Half a potato, some tuna and plenty of salad would make a much better combination.

For more detailed information on the glycemic load, refer to Patrick Holford's books: The low-GL Diet Bible and the Holford low-GL Diet Cookbook (see Resources on page 108).

P O W E R Energising Vegetables & Fruit

Pound for pound, vegetables and fruit contain far more nutrients than whole grains, so if you're looking for long-lasting energy these are a very important part of your meal.

"Eat a rainbow"

Vegetables and fruit contain a multitude of phytochemicals (phyto=plant) and antioxidants which protect your cells from 'oxidants' or free radicals (see Glossary on page 109) which can damage your health, if left unchecked. The different colours in your fruit and veg represent different phytochemicals and antioxidants so aim to 'eat the rainbow' in order to gain maximum benefit from these super healthy nutrients.

Here are just some of the wonderful vegetables and fruits you need to eat every day. Choose a 'rainbow' of colours from the following:

- **Non-starchy vegetables**: artichoke, aubergine, avocado, broccoli, cabbage, cauliflower, celeriac, celery, courgette, cucumber, fennel, garlic, green beans, kale, lettuce, mangetout, mushrooms, olives, pepper, radish, red onion, rocket, spinach, spring onion, sugar snaps, tomatoes, watercress

- **Energising fruit**: apple, apricots, blueberries, cherries, figs, grapefruit, kiwi, melon, lemons, limes, orange, papaya, peach, pear, plums, pomegranate, raspberries, strawberries

Vegetable and fruit portions

Due to their low sugar content, vegetables provide a wealth of energy nutrients without the downside of the sugar that can cause an energy slump. So there really is no limit on these and they should constitute around a third of your meal.

Fruit, on the other hand, although very nutritious does need to be limited due to its sugar content (fructose) and two portions of fruit are sufficient to keep you energised without upsetting blood sugar balance. Avoid eating too many of the very sweet fruits such as pineapple, mango, grapes and bananas and enjoy two portions of the following instead.

1 punnet of blueberries	1 punnet of strawberries
1 punnet of raspberries	1 punnet of cherries
4 apricots	4 plums
1 apple	1 kiwi
1 pear	1 orange
1 peach	Half a grapefruit
Half a papaya	Slice of watermelon

Go for 8-a-day

'5-a-day' is the government's recommendation for fruit and vegetables in the UK - but you can do better than that! Why not aim for six vegetables plus two portions of fruits?

For example, you could have tomatoes and mushrooms with scrambled eggs for breakfast. For lunch, a salad with cucumber, lettuce and avocado; some blueberries for your snack; then broccoli and beans with your main meal – simple! They can also be added to salads, soups, stuffed into your pitta breads or wraps – so no excuses!

Sprouts such as alfalfa and broccoli make a very nutritious addition to salads and wraps. You can sprout your own (see Resources on page 106) or buy them from some supermarkets or health food stores.

What about dried fruit?

Dried apricots, dates, figs, cranberries, raisins etc. have had their water removed, resulting in a high concentration of sugar. Best therefore to limit these to three or four of the larger pieces and 10-15 of the smaller piece and always consume with a few nuts and seeds for longer lasting sustenance.

P O W E R Revitalising Drinks

To maintain good energy levels and stay mentally sharp and focused, it is imperative that you stay well hydrated throughout the day. There are many drinks you can enjoy which can help keep you energised during your working day.

Water

Our bodies are comprised of 70% water, which is vital for digestion, circulation and excretion and helps carry nutrients and oxygen around the body. If you're feeling sluggish, it may be that you're dehydrated as fatigue is a common symptom of dehydration. Aim for at least 1½ litres per day, more if you're exercising, and keep a water bottle by your desk. Water can be drunk in a variety of ways:

> *Top tips:*
>
> *Fill up a 1.5 litre bottle with water (preferably filtered) at the beginning of the day and make sure it's empty by the time you go home*
>
> *Wake up with a slice of lemon and/or ginger in warm water*
>
> *Add a slice of lemon or lime to sparkling water*
>
> *It is easy to mistake thirst for hunger so if you're feeling peckish, drink a glass of water and then decide if you actually need to eat.*
>
> *Enjoy coconut water (unsweetened) for a super hydrating, healthy drink*

Juices

As these are very sweet and contain no fibre they can still cause a blood sugar spike and leave you feeling tired. So limit to one fruit juice a day, which counts as a portion of fruit. To lower the sugar content, juices are best diluted and enjoyed with some nuts to keep blood sugar balanced. Vegetable juices such as tomato, carrot or beetroot are also very sweet so limit these to just one a day.

- Fruit juices (ideally fresh or not from concentrate) e.g. orange, apple,
- Vegetable juices e.g. tomato, beetroot, carrot
- Best diluted 50/50 with water to keep blood sugar stable

Smoothies

These are a more satisfying option than juices as they include the fibre of the fruit or vegetable and can also be mixed with ground nuts or seeds to make them more filling. (See smoothie recipes on page 93). Avoid mango and pineapple as they are very sweet.

- Fruit smoothie e.g. strawberries, blueberries
- Vegetable smoothie e.g. spinach, kale, cucumber, avocado

Herbal teas and infusions

There are loads of herbals to choose from and they can all keep you refreshed and hydrated. Try any of these:

- Peppermint, rooibos (redbush), chamomile, fennel, nettle, liquorice.

Green and white tea

Green and white teas, as previously noted, are lower in caffeine than black tea and contain high amounts of the amino acid l-theanine which has a calming effect. Rich in antioxidants, these teas are associated with many health benefits including reducing the risk of heart disease.

Matcha tea - this is green tea ground into a powder and contains a much higher concentration of nutrients and antioxidants than you'll find in regular green tea bags. Limit to one a day, preferably in the early part of the day so you're sure there's no caffeine in your system at bedtime.

Coffee substitutes

Roasted Dandelion root or chicory based drinks are caffeine-free and have a similar consistency to coffee. They are popular with many of my clients and can be purchased from a good health food store. For example, 'No Caf', 'Barley Cup', Dandelion Root Coffee (Cotswold Health).

Dairy-free milk alternatives

If you have an intolerance to dairy or you prefer not to drink it, there are many dairy-free alternative 'milks' available such as oat, almond, coconut and organic soya.

What about decaffeinated drinks?

Decaffeinated tea and coffee may still contain traces of caffeine but what's more important is to go for organic and fair trade brands such as Clipper, where the caffeine is extracted naturally using carbon filtration (Swiss water process) and there are no chemical residues. Avoid brands where the caffeine is extracted using solvents as the cocktail of chemicals can be worse than the caffeine itself!

Drinks to avoid or limit

🚫 Soft drinks, juice drinks, energy drinks, alcohol and caffeine

You'll find that soft drinks and juice drinks are laden with sugar and that so-called 'energy drinks' also contain high amounts of caffeine. Whilst these drinks may cause a temporary spike in energy and alertness, you're extremely likely to come down with a crash soon afterwards.

Alcohol during your working day will make you drowsy so it goes without saying that this is not advisable if you desire to stay alert and productive. If you like to enjoy the occasional glass in the evening be aware that wine is high in sugar and registers high on the GL scale. For example, a small glass of wine is equivalent to eating a small handful of grapes so blood sugar will rise quite rapidly and then plummet. Again, follow the rule of thumb to eat some protein, such as a few nuts or some vegetable sticks and hummus with your alcoholic drink and avoid drinking it on its own.

As for tea and coffee and their inherent caffeine, I think I've said enough in the previous chapter but it's worth repeating that for sustained energy, NO caffeine is required!

So there you have it, five simple elements for an energy-filled day.

How can I sweeten my food and drinks?

Instead of sugar, there are a number of sweeteners you can use to satisfy your sweet tooth, although in time you will start to enjoy the natural sweetness from your food without needing to add more. So use these options sparingly as they can still encourage a sweet tooth if eaten in excess.

- Maple syrup, acacia honey, agave nectar, xylitol, Sweet Freedom.

- You can also use herbs, spices and juices to add natural sweetness to your foods e.g. cinnamon, nutmeg, coriander, lemon, lime, pomegranate juice.

POWER Vitamins and Minerals

By now you'll hopefully have realised that the energy drainers described in the previous chapter have very little nutrition to keep you going whilst POWER foods, which are rich in nutrients, are all critical to the energy production process. The protein, fats and carbohydrates on your POWER plate are known as *macronutrients* and they can only work effectively in the body with the help of *micronutrients*, namely vitamins and minerals.

Hundreds of chemical reactions take place before food energy (glucose) is converted to ATP, the energy the body can use, and whilst nearly all nutrients play a role in this metabolic process, some are more prevalent than others. Vitamins and minerals must be obtained from the diet as we cannot make them ourselves so let's take a look at some of these brain-boosting nutrients that can power you through your day.

B-Complex vitamins

There are nine B vitamins which work together as a complex. They are: B1 (thiamine), B2 (riboflavin), B3 (niacin), B5 (pantothenic acid), B6 (pyridoxine), B7 (biotin), B9 (folic acid), B12 (cobalamin) and choline. These B vitamins are often found in the same foods and together they help the body to use carbohydrates, proteins and fats as fuel. B vitamins are water soluble so you need to get them from your food every day.

Good sources include whole grains (B vitamins are concentrated in the bran), brewer's yeast (Marmite), brown rice, oats, nuts, wheat bran, cereals, soya, legumes, pulses, dairy products, eggs, bread, meat, poultry, fish, leafy green vegetables (e.g. kale, watercress, chard) and potatoes.

B12 is found only in animal products, so vegans often need B12 supplements, unless they are eating foods fortified with B12. Low levels of B12 can cause anaemia, and many people have trouble absorbing B12 as they get older, so deficiency can cause fatigue.

Biotin is necessary for the breakdown of fat into energy and is found in liver, fish, egg yolk, nuts, sweet potato, Swiss chard, tomatoes, carrots and avocado.

Choline is the basic building block for acetylcholine, the neurotransmitter for memory, clear thinking and concentration. It is found in egg yolks, lecithin, legumes, milk, soybeans, wholegrain cereals, chicken, sardines, turkey, cauliflower, flaxseeds, lentils and oats.

Vitamin C

Working alongside the B vitamins, vitamin C plays an important part in turning glucose into energy and is known for improving immune function and warding off coughs and colds. It is also the main ingredient in the manufacture of adrenaline and cortisol in the adrenal glands, together with B5, so it can help alleviate stress. Like the B vitamins, vitamin C is water soluble so needs to be topped up regularly.

Vitamin C is found in all fresh fruit and vegetables, particularly all citrus fruits, kiwi, goji berries, blueberries, strawberries, blackcurrants, acerola cherries, cantaloupe melons, pineapples, peppers, sweet potatoes and dark green leafy vegetables such as kale.

Magnesium

Magnesium is required for many cellular functions, especially the production of energy. Known as 'nature's tranquiliser' it can help reduce stress and anxiety, and aid sleep. Magnesium occurs abundantly in natural, unprocessed foods so consuming large amounts of processed, refined foods could make you deficient in this important mineral. Best dietary sources include legumes, nuts, seeds, whole grains, tofu and green leafy vegetables. Avoid overcooking foods to minimise loss of magnesium.

Iron

Iron plays an essential role in metabolism and therefore an important mineral for healthy energy levels. It forms part of haemoglobin in your red blood cells, necessary for carrying oxygen around the body. Iron deficiency can lead to anaemia, leaving you tired and susceptible to illness. Good sources of iron include organic red meat, chicken, liver, eggs, fish and plant sources include legumes such as soybeans, lentils and chickpeas, whole grains, nuts, seeds and green leafy vegetables. Vitamin C aids the absorption of iron so eating fruit alongside your iron-rich food is recommended, for example an orange with your boiled egg.

Chromium

Chromium works closely with insulin, helping it direct glucose into the cells and is a key player in blood sugar control, helping your body process sugar. Lost in processed foods, it is found in liver, egg yolks, cheese, poultry, shellfish, broccoli, whole grains, pulses and spices, nuts, wheat germ, brewer's yeast, fruit and juices, mushrooms, asparagus.

Zinc

Zinc is also required to produce insulin and to regulate blood sugar. It plays a role in energy production so we need it to keep energy levels high.

It's found in sea foods especially oysters, shellfish, canned fish, lean red meat, green leafy vegetables, mushrooms, potatoes, nuts especially pecans, seeds especially pumpkin, cereals, rice, rye, oats, lentils, pulses, whole grains, cheese, wholemeal bread and eggs.

Calcium

Whilst associated primarily with bone health, calcium is also required for metabolism and energy production.

Found in milk, cheese, eggs, fortified bread, canned fish especially salmon, nuts, seeds, dark green leafy vegetables, parsley, cabbage, root vegetables and blackstrap molasses.

The importance of fibre

Whilst fibre is not a nutrient, as it isn't absorbed by the body, it is a very important part of these whole foods. Fibre comes in soluble and insoluble forms both of which confer different health benefits:

Soluble fibre, found in beans and lentils, oats, pulses and fruit, slows down the release of sugar into your blood and can actually decrease the glycemic load of your meal, giving you longer lasting energy. It is also linked with lowering cholesterol and a reduced risk of diabetes.

Insoluble fibre helps prevent constipation so is important for a healthy bowel. Good sources include wholegrain and wholemeal bread, brown rice, fruit and vegetables, nuts and seeds. It is also present in whole grain breakfast cereals but I do not recommend these as they are processed and often contain added sugar.

The recommended amount of fibre per adult is 18g per day and if you follow the POWER plan you will be getting plenty.

Co-enzyme Q10

CoQ10 is a vitamin-like substance found in most cells, particularly the mitochondria, the 'powerhouses' that generate most of the cells' energy. Although it's made in the body, it can also be found in food, particularly fish, meat and poultry, but small amounts are in nuts, seeds and beans. CoQ10 levels decrease with age and it can be taken in supplement form (see Resources on page 106).

Energy supplements

Sometimes, with the best will in the world, you still may find your energy flagging. Don't despair as many of the above nutrients can be found as supplements and there are a number of herbs too that can help with energy and stress. Here are some ideas but please seek advice from a nutritional expert who will assess your needs.

- Take a good quality multivitamin and mineral supplement that delivers all the nutrients, including the B complex 'energy' vitamins that can address any shortfall in your diet.

- Vitamin C - helps support your adrenals and your immune system, keeping stress levels down and bugs at bay.

- Fish oils – essential role in cellular energy production

- Other supplements and herbs: CoQ10, Ginseng, Rhodiola rosea, Ginkgo Biloba.

Caution: these may be contraindicated with certain drugs so seek advice from a health professional if you are taking medication.

For details of where to buy supplements, see Resources page 106.

So now you know all about my POWER Eating Programme™ and I hope you feel ready to start enjoying these wholesome, delicious foods and feeling your energy levels soar!

Before you read on here's a quick round up of my favourite POWER foods:

Top POWER foods and drinks
Avocado · Berries
Coconut · Eggs
Garlic · Green leafy vegetables
Lemon · Nuts
Oats · Oily fish
Quinoa · Seeds
WATER

.

Chapter 3: POWER Meal Solutions

In this chapter I have created a series of energy-boosting meal solutions to make it easy for you to follow my POWER Eating Programme™. The following meal options cater for all tastes and situations – whether you're making your own, buying from a sandwich bar or supermarket or eating in the office restaurant.

POWER Check

What to include	How many meals per day
Protein	Every meal
Oils & Fats	At least two
Whole Grains & Starches	At least two
Energising Veg & Fruit	At least three
Revitalising drinks	Throughout the day

My suggestions are realistic and practical, as well as healthy, to fit in with your lifestyle and to keep you on track. Although I've listed meals in the conventional order of breakfast, lunch and snacks, there's nothing to stop you from switching them around. After all, in Asia you'll find noodles or curry on the breakfast menu and in Mediterranean countries salads are commonly eaten for breakfast. So if you're feeling peckish in the afternoon, have some muesli, and if you only have time for yoghurt with some seeds and berries for lunch, that's so much better than nothing at all.

Furthermore, if you find yourself eating the same foods every day initially that's absolutely fine. As I say: "Repetition is better than poor nutrition".

Each meal type shows an example of a POWER meal. For more suggestions, simply go to **www.nocaffeinerequired.com** and you'll be assembling your own POWER meals in no time.

POWER breakfasts

If you start the day with a wholesome, nutritious breakfast, you are much more likely to continue to eat the right foods for the rest of the day. However, the opposite is also true and many of my clients who either skip breakfast or choose some fast releasing sugary cereal will undoubtedly yo-yo through their day and plummet predictably into that mid-afternoon slump.

Remember that if you skip breakfast, your blood sugar will be very low after several hours without food. By the time you get into the office you are likely to go for the wrong food just to get your ever diminishing energy levels up again. So start as you mean to go on and have a satiating, energising breakfast from the outset.

If you don't like to eat first thing or you simply don't have time, then have a revitalising warm lemon water to kick-start your liver into action and stimulate your digestive juices. You can then eat breakfast a little while later, or even on the way to work. If you do stop off at a coffee shop, consider something other than a coffee – a green tea for example has less caffeine and gives the system a light boost rather than a jolt.

Cereal-based breakfasts

Oat-based cereals are the best choice as they release energy slowly e.g. muesli, granola, porridge, breakfast cookies (see recipes on pages 83-88). Wheat-based cereals e.g. Weetabix are more processed than oats but if you want them, be sure to add the extra POWER components.

Porridge	P	O	W	E	R
Oats		•			
Milk	•				
Grated apple with cinnamon			•		
Seeds	•	•			
Warm ginger & lemon water					•

Bread- and cracker-based breakfasts

Toast and jam is basically sugar and starch, so there are far better options to kick start your day. Ideally, have one or two slices of bread per day and the rest of the time go for the oatcakes and crackers.

Smoked salmon on toast	P	O	W	E	R
Rye, sourdough or wholegrain toast			•		
Smoked salmon	•	•			
Cucumber and cherry tomatoes				•	
Toasted pumpkin seeds	•	•			
Lemon water					•

Egg-based breakfasts

Eggs are a great source of protein so will really fill you up. Go for two rather than just one to make it more substantial. To improve the uptake of the iron from the eggs, include a source of vitamin C with your meal e.g. fruit, veg or juices. Ideal for breakfast, lunch and snacks.

Scrambled eggs on toast	P	O	W	E	R
2 scrambled eggs made with butter / coconut oil	•	•			
Smoked salmon	•				
Cherry tomatoes				•	
Wholemeal toast or pitta (optional)			•		
Glass of fresh orange juice					•

Yoghurts

Yoghurt can be eaten for breakfast, lunch, snacks and makes a healthy dessert. Low-fat is ok but full-fat will keep you fuller for longer and don't even think about fat-free! Goat's or Sheep's milk yoghurt can be easier on the digestion and soya yoghurt (unflavoured and unsweetened) is a good dairy-free option.

Coconut yoghurt (Co-Yo) is delicious and becoming more widely available. Fruit adds enough sweetness to the yogurt, in my opinion, but if you 'need' extra sweetness add a drizzle of acacia honey, maple or agave syrup.

Fruit salad and yoghurt	P	O	W	E	R
Small pot of natural live yoghurt	•				
Kiwi, strawberries, blueberries				•	
2 tsp of ground flaxseeds or chia seeds	•	•			
Quinoa (optional)	•		•		
Glass of water					•

Smoothies and Juices

Fantastically revitalising, a smoothie can be a whole meal in a glass provided each POWER component is present. Great for breakfast or in the afternoon as an instant pick-me-up. You'll need a good blender to whiz this all up (see recipes on page 93).

High energy berry smoothie	P	O	W	E	R
Mixed berries and half a banana				•	
Yoghurt and / or milk	•				
Ground flaxseeds and almonds	•	•			
Soaked oats (optional)				•	
Water or coconut water					•

Top tip:

If you prefer not to put nuts or seeds in the smoothie, you can eat a handful afterwards to avoid a blood sugar spike / dip

POWER lunches

It is 1 pm and you've been beavering away all morning and suddenly you're ravenous but you haven't a clue what you're going to eat. So you hotfoot it to the nearest sandwich bar or vending machine, wolf down a sandwich and a packet of crisps - probably at your desk – then, temporarily satisfied, start to deal with the next email. Over time, this type of behaviour will take its toll on your energy, your waistline and your overall wellbeing.

If this is a fairly accurate assessment of your lunch 'hour', you're not alone because on average, according to a survey of 2,000 full-time workers by OnePoll (2013), we take less than half an hour for lunch as we are too busy.

Jobs can be stressful and very demanding on your mind and body. So make sure you're prepared for those demands by choosing a healthy lunch that can help boost your energy for the rest of the day, without having to resort to stimulants galore to stay awake. Choose your lunches carefully from the following options and keep a food diary to see which foods energise and which drain you.

Bread-based lunches

Too much bread, especially wheat-based, can make you drowsy in the afternoon so stick to the recommended quantities e.g. an open sandwich rather than two slices of bread to keep you energised. Experiment with different toppings and fillings.

Chicken and salad wrap / sandwich	P	O	W	E	R
Wholemeal wrap / pitta bread			•		
Chicken pieces	•	•			
Non-starchy salad vegetables				•	
Avocado	•				
Olive oil based dressing		•			
Peppermint tea					•

> *Top tip:*
>
> *To reduce the amount of bread you can replace the top slice with an iceberg or Cos lettuce leaf to keep the contents in. Or you can have a 'breadless' sandwich and use lettuce leaves instead of bread.*

POWER salads

Prepare your salad the night before for a truly energising lunch. There are many ready-made options too but as always make sure they contain all the right POWER components.

Tuna Niçoise	P	O	W	E	R
Tuna – fresh or tinned and hardboiled egg	•				
Green beans, tomatoes, lettuce				•	
White or sweet potato			•		
Olives		•		•	
Dressing with olive oil, lemon juice		•		•	
Redbush (rooibos) tea					•

POWER soups

Soups are a fantastic way of incorporating all your POWER ingredients into one bowl or mug. When buying soups make sure you've always got the protein like chicken, ham or beans (see below). No need for bread as there's already enough starch in the soup. Avoid soups that contain only vegetables such as carrot and coriander or tomato soup as these will not fill you up.

Leek, bean and potato soup	P	O	W	E	R
Cannelini beans	•				
Leek, garlic				•	
Potatoes / carrots (small amounts)			•		
Coconut or olive oil		•			
Water					•

Egg-based lunches

Similar to breakfast ideas but you may want to incorporate more salad / non-starchy vegetables and meats at lunchtime. I'm not a fan of a standard shop-bought egg mayo sandwich as there's too much bread and too much 'bad fat' mayo so avoid if possible. Notice there are no whole grains or starches (W) in the lunch option below and you may feel more energised without them provided you eat plenty of energising veg.

Mushroom omelette	P	O	W	E	R
Eggs	•				
Butter, coconut or olive oil		•			
Mushrooms				•	
Green leafy salad				•	
Pomegranate juice diluted with water					•

Hot lunches

If you're lucky enough to have a restaurant at work, or if you eat out, make sure you are making the right choices. You can of course reheat leftovers from the night before and there are some very effective food flasks that will keep your stews and soups hot for 5-6 hours (see Resources on page 106). If you like to use a microwave to reheat your food, avoid using plastic containers especially for fatty food such as meats and cheeses, as the very high temperatures may cause harmful chemicals to seep out of the plastic and into the food. Use a glass or ceramic container instead that you can store in the office kitchen.

Grilled Salmon & vegetables	P	O	W	E	R
Salmon fillet	•	•			
Potatoes (max 3 small)			•		
Broccoli, beans, courgettes				•	
Lemon and ginger herbal tea					•

POWER snacks

Never again will you feel restricted to a biscuit and a cup of tea! The options are endless here and provided you go for a bit of protein for continued sustenance you can vary the components to suit. Many snacks are ideal to have in your bag or the car when you're on the run so make sure you've always got a good stock of the essentials.

Oatcakes, nut butter & berries	P	O	W	E	R
2 or 3 oatcakes			•		
Almond or hazelnut butter	•	•			
Blueberries			•		
White tea with vanilla					•

Evening meals

Your plan will also need to include evening meals as these are equally important to keep your energy levels steady for the following day. After all, there's no point in coming home to a plate of chips and a couple of pints of beer and then expecting to feel good the following day! Here's an example of how to keep the POWER going in the evening.

Chicken stir-fry with brown rice	P	O	W	E	R
Chicken fillet	•	•			
30 g of brown basmati rice			•		
Red pepper, bean sprouts, mushrooms, cabbage, leeks				•	
Peppermint tea					•

So you've seen that there is a multitude of options that will keep your energy flowing smoothly throughout the day. For more inspiring ideas, take a look at **www.nocaffeinerequired.com**.

The next chapter will help you plan your POWER meals.

Chapter 4: Planning your POWER Meals

"If you fail to plan, you plan to fail". I can't emphasise the importance of planning enough and when my clients find themselves making the wrong food choices, they admit that it's generally due to lack of planning.

So this chapter helps you get organised so that you always have what you need to stay powered up. Whether you're working from home or in the office, planning is simply giving some thought to something very important in your life, namely the way you choose to nourish yourself. It makes no difference whether you're packing your own lunch box, eating in the staff restaurant, having breakfast at your desk or buying from a sandwich bar – you just need to know you've got all the right ingredients to ride smoothly through your day.

Benefits of planning:

- Ensures you are eating healthier, better-balanced and more energising foods

- Saves you time

- Stops you making the wrong choices or overeating

- Cheaper than ready-made options if you've made foods yourself

- Keeps waste to a minimum as you'll have what you need

- Prevents 'snack attacks'

- Knowing what you're going to eat during the week can also reduce stress – at least you won't be worrying about what you're going to eat.

Making time

Never enough time? If you think you don't have time to plan, think again and ask yourself whether good health, high energy and wellbeing are a worthwhile investment. Once you discover the benefits of the POWER Eating Programme™, you'll never want to be without any of your energy-boosting foods again. You'll want to find time to plan, shop and prepare and what's more, you'll see that planning doesn't take long at all once you get into the habit.

Getting started

When you plan you need to ask yourself these questions:

When is the best time to plan for the week ahead?

Meal planning should be treated like any other important appointment in your diary so the first thing to consider is when to plan. For example, Sunday could be the ideal time to plan your week's meals so you've got what you need both at home and at work to stay powered up.

What am I going to eat?

Before you make a plan, make sure you've read the previous chapters so that you're clear about what you need to eat for optimum energy and vitality. Then make a list of the meals and snacks that would suit your taste and lifestyle. Even if you don't have time to prepare your own meals, your planner could still include what you intend to eat from your local salad bar or office restaurant.

POWER switches – what can I change right now?

Go to **www.nocaffeinerequired.com** and download the POWER Switch Sheet. Write down what you are currently eating in the first column and the more energising alternatives in the second. Below are some simple switches you can make immediately without having to spend hours on a complicated plan and you'll see how just a few changes can make a big difference to your energy and wellbeing.

Instead of:	Switch to:
Cornflakes	Porridge / Muesli

Instead of:	Switch to:
Tuna baguette	Tuna in wholemeal pitta and salad
Margarine	Butter, coconut oil, tahini, drizzle of olive oil
Sausage roll	2 slices of turkey on rye bread
Kitkat	2 or 3 cubes of dark chocolate
Biscuits	Oatcake with nut butter
Crisps	Oaty bakes / nuts / vegetable crisps (occasionally)
Coffee	Barley Cup / No Caf / Dandelion root
Tea	Herbal teas / water with lemon and ginger

Where am I going to get it from?

Whether you're making your own or buying ready-made foods, you'll need to know the best places to source your POWER food. Apart from the obvious food outlets you may want to consider buying fresh, seasonal produce from your local farmers' market. Alternatively, think about delivery companies such as Abel & Cole or Riverford for organic produce including fruit, vegetables, meats, fish and cheese (see Resources on page 106).

Maybe consider clubbing together with some colleagues from the office to buy your POWER food in bulk!

What will I need to transport my food?

Depending on whether your food will be eaten hot or cold, you'll need to purchase insulated cooler bags, ice packs, thermos flasks and water bottles (see Resources on page 106).

Write your plan

If you write something down you're much more likely to stick to it. So go to **www.nocaffeinerequired.com,** download the POWER Meal Planner and jot down the meals you intend to eat for the forthcoming week (see sample plan on page 57). Tick the POWER checklist each time so you're sure all the right components are there. Either print or save to 'cloud' so that it's accessible whenever you want it.

Bonus: POWER Meal Plan

Go to www.nocaffeinerequired.com & sign up for your free menu plan

---

Food diary

Some of my clients use their food diary to double up as a planner, so not only can they see what they intend to eat during the week but they can also keep track of what they've eaten.

Bonus: FREE* 5-Day Food Diary Review

Download the *POWER Food & Energy diary from* www.nocaffeinerequired.com. Write down your food intake for 5 days then return to info@nocaffeinerequired.com for FREE analysis and feedback on your food choices. * Offer limited to the first 100 applicants

---

Make a list

Bonus: FREE POWER Shopping List

Download the free shopping list *from* www.nocaffeinerequired.com. The POWER Shopping List will be kept updated, including new items and recommended brands that will keep your meals interesting, tasty and energising. Make sure you add them to your favourites if shopping online.

POWER staples

Make sure you've always got these items in your cupboard and freezer so that even if you've run out of fresh food you can still throw something nutritious together that will supply the energy you need. It's actually rather satisfying to open a tin of tuna, cook up a bit of pasta and use up any vegetables that have been sitting in the fridge. So if you have these essentials in your cupboard, you can't go far wrong. Below is a list of staples to get you started.

Protein options

- Tinned tuna, salmon, anchovies, herring

- Tinned artichokes, asparagus, hearts of palm, sweetcorn

- Tinned beans – cannellini, kidney, haricot, butterbean, aduki, mixed beans, baked beans

Oils & Fats

- Coconut oil, extra virgin olive oil, flax oil

- Pack or jar of olives

- Packs of nuts – walnuts, almonds, pecans, hazelnuts, cashews, brazils

- Packs of seeds – flaxseeds, sunflower, pumpkin, sesame seeds

- Coconut milk

- Jar of tahini (sesame paste)

- Nut butters - almond / hazelnut / peanut

Whole grains and starchy options

- Wholemeal pasta, brown rice, quinoa, wholemeal couscous, barley

- Oatcakes, Ryvita

- Packs of ready cooked quinoa, brown rice

- Soba noodles

- Frozen bread and wraps

Energising vegetables and fruit

- Tinned tomatoes, sun dried tomatoes, passata, tomato purée
- Tinned peaches, apricots, pineapple
- Jar of pesto
- Dried apricots (best: organic, no sulphur), dried figs, raisins, goji berries
- Bottle of lemon juice
- Frozen berries
- Frozen peas, broccoli, beans
- Apple juice (ideally not made from concentrate)
- Frozen chopped onions

Revitalising drinks

- Water – ideally filtered. If you buy bottled water, store in a cool place.
- Coconut water
- Herbal teas: rooibos, peppermint, camomile, fennel
- Coffee substitutes: Barley Cup, Dandelion root

Stocks and flavourings

- Tamari, soy sauce or Bragg's aminos for flavourings
- Vinegars e.g. apple cider, balsamic
- Sauces – e.g. low sugar and salt pasta sauces
- Harissa paste

On the next page is a sample weekly POWER menu plan and you'll find plenty more ideas on **www.nocaffeinerequired.com** and on my Facebook page **No Caffeine Required**.

Sample Weekly POWER Menu Plan

Monday		P	O	W	E	R
Breakfast	Homemade muesli	✓	✓	✓	✓	
Snack	Apple + small handful of almonds	✓	✓		✓	
Lunch	Chicken, quinoa + vegetable soup	✓			✓	
Snack	2 oatcakes + celery sticks with hummus	✓	✓	✓	✓	
Drinks	Hot water & lemon, peppermint tea, water					✓
Dinner	Chicken stir fry with brown rice, vegetables	✓	✓	✓	✓	

Tuesday						
Breakfast	Scrambled eggs, w/meal toast, grilled tomatoes. Half a grapefruit.	✓	✓	✓	✓	
Snack	2 oatcakes with nut butter e.g. almond or peanut	✓	✓	✓		
Lunch	Salade Niçoise – tuna, boiled egg, green beans, salad, olives, 2 small potatoes	✓	✓	✓	✓	
Snack	6 cubes of feta with 6 olives and pumpkin seeds.	✓	✓		✓	
Drinks	Water, liquorice tea, green tea					✓
Dinner	Salmon teriyaki, broccoli, tomatoes, 3 new potatoes	✓	✓	✓	✓	

Wednesday						
Breakfast	Porridge, grated apple, cinnamon, flaxseed	✓	✓	✓	✓	
Snack	2 squares dark chocolate with 2 Brazil nuts	✓	✓			
Lunch	Vegetable and herb tortilla + green salad	✓	✓		✓	
Snack	Yoghurt with seeds and berries				✓	
Drinks	Water, peppermint tea, coconut water					✓
Dinner	Chilli bean casserole with quinoa and green veg	✓	✓	✓	✓	

Thursday						
Breakfast	Breakfast Smoothie	✓	✓	✓	✓	
Snack	Peach and 5 walnuts	✓	✓		✓	
Lunch	Tuna or chilli bean wrap with avocado and salad	✓	✓	✓	✓	
Snack	2 oatcakes with mackerel pâté	✓	✓	✓	✓	
Drinks	Warm lemon water, water, redbush tea					✓
Dinner	Baked beans on wholegrain toast and green salad	✓	✓	✓	✓	

Friday						
Breakfast	Low carb granola. 2 tbsp oats, yoghurt + berries	✓	✓	✓	✓	
Snack	Nut and seed bar (see Resources on page 106)	✓	✓	✓		
Lunch	Iceberg lettuce 'sandwich' with prawns and salad	✓	✓		✓	
Snack	Celery sticks filled with almond / peanut butter	✓	✓		✓	
Drinks	Water, nettle tea, chamomile tea, decaf coffee					✓
Dinner	Spaghetti bolognaise, loads of veg, a little pasta	✓		✓	✓	

Go to **www.nocaffeinerequired.com** for more menu plans

Chapter 5: Smart Ways to Execute your POWER Plan

In this chapter I share with you some smart ideas for preparing your meals, either from scratch or throwing some healthy convenience foods together. Again, even if you're the 'grab and go' type, you'll find out what the best choices are and where to source them.

Food prep ideas that save you time and money

Depending on your plan and how much time you have available, there may be a number of things you need to prepare at the beginning of the week. This may involve making up salads or sandwiches the night before or simply making sure you've got a stash of nuts, oatcakes, fruit and water for your desk. A bit of preparation can save you time, money and stress during your busy day.

Practical, realistic and convenient

I'd like these ideas to be practical and realistic so rather than worry about the lost nutrients in pre-cut vegetable sticks, remember that it's much better to eat vegetables instead of crisps for your snack. Also, it may be more cost-effective if it means you'll actually eat them. Of course you don't have to make something for every day of the week – you could plan to make a soup that you'll have on two days, sandwich-based meals on another two days and on one day you may want to treat yourself to a ready-made salad where you don't have to lift a finger.

Preparation aids

If you intend to make your meals from scratch there are a number of essential items you'll need for the plan to work efficiently.

- Food processor for whizzing up dips and sauces, chopping and grating vegetables
- Blender for soups and smoothies

- Hand held 'stick' blender for soups

- Plastic storage containers and bags for transporting your food to work (see Resources on page 106)

- Microwave-safe containers. Many office kitchens are equipped with a microwave and although not the best way of cooking as nutrients are lost, it is highly convenient and means you can heat up anything from soups to veg pots to porridge. Ideally use glass or ceramic cooking containers rather than plastic.

- Use non-pvc cling film to wrap your foods

Batch cooking

If you have a couple of hours to spare at the weekend, why not make a big box of muesli, a couple of batches of breakfast cookies, a few fillets of poached salmon or chicken or a vat of soup? Most foods will keep for at least 2-3 days in the fridge and if you're not planning on using them immediately they'll keep in the freezer for 3 months.

Using leftovers

Put anything left over from the evening meal such as vegetables, rice, quinoa, chicken, beef, stir-fried veg into an air-tight container (see Resources on page 106), pop into the fridge then that's your next day's lunch sorted. Any leftovers can be frozen so make sure you make a double or triple batch.

Plan your leftovers!

Rather than leaving it to chance and hoping there'll be something left over after the evening meal, plan to make a bit extra, such as an extra chicken fillet. This can go straight into the lunch box for the following day.

Freezing

Make friends with your freezer as this can be a huge time saver. You can freeze most things from bread, wraps etc, soups, vegetables, fruit and milk to meat, poultry and fish.

Storing grains

Grains, especially rice, can grow mould and bacteria very quickly if left out so as soon as they've cooled down, put any leftovers in the fridge where they can keep for three days. Add a small amount of water to the grains before reheating as they tend to dry out in the fridge, then reheat thoroughly. Alternatively, if you make a large batch of rice, divide it into smaller portions and freeze. Then all you need to do is take it out and pop it in the microwave at work until cooked through. It actually tastes freshly cooked when reheated from frozen.

Transporting hot meals

You can purchase very effective food flasks that will keep your food hot for several hours (see Resources on page 106).

Best ways to cook

In an ideal world we would all be steaming our food in order to preserve the maximum amount of nutrients, but this is not always practical with our busy lifestyles. So follow these tips to cook as effectively as possible:

- When steaming vegetables, use a steamer basket and cook until the vegetables are 'al dente' and not soggy. Cook vegetables for as little time as possible as the longer you cook them, the more nutrients will be lost.

- Poaching involves covering the food (e.g. fish, chicken) in water, milk or a light stock and simmering gently. This is a great way to infuse flavour into food.

- To poach eggs you simply add the eggs to the gently rolling water and cook for 4 minutes.

- 'Steam frying' is a healthier way of stir-frying as the oil doesn't get overheated. The vegetables are added to hot water or stock in the pan and cooked quickly until they are 'al dente'. Oil, such as olive oil, can be added at the end of cooking to prevent the oil from overheating and creating damaging molecules.

- When boiling don't cover your vegetables with water, just use as little water as possible and keep the lid on.

- Grilling food that contains fat is less damaging than frying but cook on a medium setting and ensure you don't burn it.

- If baking chicken 'parcels' in the oven use baking parchment rather than foil which can leach aluminium into your food - you can then wrap parchment in foil to secure it.

- Microwaving is thought to destroy more nutrients than steaming but again use as little water as possible so that the nutrients don't end up in the water.

- Avoid deep frying and when shallow frying use small amounts of coconut or olive oil rather than vegetable oils. Barbecuing should be kept to a minimum as burnt or charred food can produce harmful free radicals (see Glossary on page 109).

Executing your POWER plan

The following tables show you some of the key ways in which you can execute your POWER plan, giving you the option to make or buy your own food, subject to time and budget constraints.

Make

If you enjoy cooking, I have listed many foods that you can prepare from scratch for the week ahead. This can work out cheaper than buying ready-made meals, but you need to balance time with cost. Alongside these ideas, you'll find plenty of handy tips and time savers.

Buy

If you'd prefer to 'grab and run', there are plenty of healthy options you can buy off the shelf either in supermarkets or sandwich bars. Always check the 'balance of POWER' in soups, salads and wraps. Where's the protein? Plenty of vegetables? Not too much starch?

Avoid

Avoid these shop-bought foods as they will sap your energy.

POWER breakfasts in action

	Muesli
Make	• Homemade muesli mix (see recipe on page 83)
	– *Make enough to last several days*
	– *Add milk or dairy-free alternative when ready to eat*
	– *Pre-soak overnight if you like a soft consistency*
	– *Add yogurt or fresh fruit*
Buy	• Basic muesli mix - oats, nuts and seeds
	– *Add extra oats, coconut, chopped nuts, flaxseeds and fresh berries for extra POWER!*
Avoid	• Mueslis high in dried fruit, malted flakes and sugar

	Porridge
Make	• Overnight Porridge Oats (see recipe on page 84)
	– *Soak overnight in milk or dairy-free alternative*
	– *Can be eaten cold or heated on hob or in microwave*
	– *Add a few chopped nuts, seeds and berries*
	– *Make enough for 2 or 3 days*
Buy	• Ready cooked takeaway porridge from certain outlets
	– *Add chopped nuts, seeds, berries*
Avoid	• Instant porridge pots from supermarkets - very flaky and sugary - and won't sustain you!

Granola

Make • Homemade granola (see recipe on page 84)
  - *Eat as a cereal or add to yoghurt*

Buy • Low GL granola e.g. Lizi's Granola
  - *Mix with oats and extra nuts/seeds as still sweet when served 'neat'*

Avoid • Sugary, refined breakfast cereals
  • Sugary granola and cereal bars from food outlets

Healthy Baked Goods

Make • Breakfast muffins, flapjacks or cookies (see pages 86 and 87)
  - *Great as a snack or breakfast on the go.*
  - *Easy to freeze*

Buy • Nakd bars, Bounce bars, Pulsin' bars (see Resources on page 106)

Avoid • Shop bought muffins, granola, flapjacks, cereal bars

Smoothies

Make • Whiz up berries, yoghurt, juice, half banana, oats, ground nuts, protein powder (see recipes on page 93)
  - *A fantastic all-in-one POWER meal*

Buy • Smoothies made with berries e.g. Innocent
  - *Eat with some protein e.g. a few walnuts or some yoghurt to fill you up*

Avoid • Smoothies with sweet tropical fruits e.g. mango and pineapple
  • Juices and juice drinks as too sugary

POWER lunches in action

	Sandwiches
Make	• Use wholemeal, wholegrain, rye bread, wholemeal pitta and wraps, oatcakes – *Prepare fillings with protein and salad options (see below)*
Buy	• Wholemeal sandwiches or wraps with chicken / hummus / beans / egg and plenty of salad – *Eat with extra veg e.g. cherry tomatoes, pepper, radishes, lettuce to boost the POWER*
Avoid	• White bread, panini, baguettes, bagels, water crackers, rice cakes, thick mayonnaise, processed meats e.g. salami, turkey ham

	Grains
Make	• Brown rice, quinoa (see how to cook quinoa on page 86), bulgur wheat, millet, couscous, wholewheat or gluten free pasta – *Add to salads and soups* – *Mix grains with salad veg and protein (see recipe for Quinoa and mackerel salad)*
Buy	• Cooked quinoa, rice, bulgur wheat, giant couscous e.g. Merchant Gourmet, Food Doctor (see Resources on page 106) or own brands – *Eat hot or cold and add to salad and soups* – *Ready-made salads with grains e.g. quinoa or couscous with roasted vegetables and chickpeas* – *Add extra protein to ready-made if needed*
Avoid	• White pasta, noodles, pot noodles

Protein – Meat & Poultry

Make • Grill or bake (in foil) chicken fillet or poach in boiling water with stock
  - *Marinate in tamari (soy) sauce, chilli, garlic & ginger*
  - *Leftovers from roast are ideal e.g. roast beef or chicken*

Buy • Pre-cooked chicken pieces, hand carved turkey / ham
  • Wide range of ready-made wraps / sandwiches / soups and salads with chicken / duck / beef and veg is available.

Avoid • Processed meat with high salt and low meat content e.g. salami
  • Burgers and fatty sausages

Protein - Fish

Make • Grill or bake (in foil) fresh salmon, trout, cod or haddock
  • Stir fry prawns

Buy • Pre-cooked salmon, smoked salmon, mackerel or trout fillets
  • Pack of prawns, tinned salmon, tuna, sardines, mackerel, anchovies

Avoid • Prawn or tuna mayonnaise sandwiches or salads

Protein - Eggs

Make • Hard-boil for 8-10 minutes
  - *Make the night before and store in fridge*
  - *Eat for breakfast, snacks or pitta bread with some salad*
  • Vegetable frittata (see page 91)

Buy	• Ready-made Spanish tortilla
	– *Enjoy with salad*
Avoid	• Shop bought egg mayonnaise

Protein - Dairy

Make	• Cut up cubes of feta or mozzarella; grill halloumi; grate small amount of cheddar
	– *Add to salads or roasted vegetables*
	– *Mix fresh or frozen berries with natural yoghurt and top with granola*
Buy	• Cottage or cream cheese, Goat's cheese, live natural yoghurt
	– *Eat cheese with oatcakes as a snack*
Avoid	• Too much rich cheese as difficult to digest
	• Processed cheeses e.g. 'cheese strings', fruit or flavoured yoghurts, plastic tubes of fromage frais, cheesy pizza

Protein – Beans & Pulses

Make	• Lentils
	– *Cook lentils e.g. red, green or brown, for 20 minutes with some stock and use for soups, salads, dahl*
	• Beans and chickpeas
	– *Soak overnight and cook for 30-40 minutes*
	– *Use for soups, salads, wraps and dips*
Buy	• Tinned beans or lentils e.g. baked beans, cannellini, butter beans, haricot, pinto, aduki, kidney, chickpeas, Puy lentils, chilli beans
	– *Also available in pots, pouches (e.g. Merchant Gourmet) and cartons*
	• Ready to eat falafel, bean/lentil salads, bean and veg soups
	– *Veg pots e.g. Innocent, Food Doctor (see page 106)*

Avoid	• Baked beans high in sugar and salt

Protein - Tofu

Make	• Cut tofu into 1 cm cubes
	    – *Marinate tofu in tamari and spices then gently fry*
	    – *Use soft silken tofu as base for 'soyannaise' (see page 93)*

Buy	• Marinated tofu pieces (e.g. Cauldron) • Miso soup • Smoked tofu with almonds or basil tofu (Taifun) - delicious!
Avoid	• Non-organic tofu, if possible, as likely to be genetically modified

Salads

Make	• Make your own salad bowl with cherry tomatoes, celery, cucumber, grated carrot, beetroot, avocado, spinach, rocket, lettuce, watercress
	• Chop up carrots, celery and cucumber sticks
	    – *Add a squeeze of lemon juice to avocado to stop it turning brown*
	    – *Enjoy veg sticks with dips e.g. hummus*
	    – *Add to sandwiches / pitta / wraps*
	    – *Add dressing just before eating to prevent going soggy*

Buy	• Pre-washed leaves, salad bags or salad bowls
	    – *Add protein e.g. prawns, anchovies, tuna, chicken, beans, chickpeas, egg*
	    – *Pre-cut veg sticks*
	    – *Ready-made salads e.g. 3-bean, tuna Niçoise*
	    – *Remember: run a POWER check before you buy!*

Avoid	• Ready-made salads such as coleslaw and potato salad loaded with mayonnaise

Soups

Make • Cook hearty soups with plenty of non-starchy vegetables and protein such as beans, lentils, quinoa, chicken, ham, bacon (see page 92)
- *Make a large batch and store in fridge for up to 3 days or freeze*
- *Can be heated and stored in good thermos for up to 5 hours*

Buy • Fresh or tinned soups
- *Add chicken, tofu, beans, quinoa, chickpeas to a vegetable soup for extra protein and fibre if necessary*

Avoid • Vegetable-only soups such as carrot & coriander or tomato soup - no protein so they won't fill you up
• Creamy soups, 'Cup-a-Soup'

POWER snacks in action

Nuts & Seeds

Make • Toast almonds in oven on low heat for 15 minutes
• Chop almonds, walnuts and pecans for muesli or toppings
• Make up a trail mix (see page 95) and put some into a small container the night before
• Dry fry sunflower / pumpkin seeds until lightly toasted
• Nut butters e.g. cashew, almond, peanuts (use powerful blender)
- *Always keep a stash of nuts & seeds with you and eat any time of day – even on the way to work if you're in a rush!*

Buy • Packs of raw, unsalted nuts
• Toasted seeds in soy sauce (e.g. Food Doctor, Munchy Seeds)
• Trail mix

	• Peanut butter (low salt, sugar-free), almond, hazelnut, cashew butters
Avoid	• Salted, honey roasted nuts
	• Salty, sugary peanut butter with bad fats

Dips

Make	• Homemade dips e.g. pesto, hummus (see recipe on page 88, aubergine, bean dips, guacamole
	   – *Quick to make and healthier than shop bought*
	   – *Eat with raw celery, carrot, cucumber sticks*

Buy	• Readymade dips and pots of hummus
	   – *Add your own chickpeas or pine nuts for extra POWER*
	   – *Look for dips that contain olive oil*

Avoid	• Cheap dips such as tarasamalata and economy priced hummus as full of bad fats

More Ready-to-Eat Options

Buy	• Edamame beans • Fresh coconut pieces • Fresh fruit salad • Oatcakes • Dr Karg spelt crackers • Oaty bakes (Nairns) • Dried apricots (always consume with nuts or seeds)
Avoid	• Crisps, pretzels, rice crackers • Chocolates, biscuits, cakes, cereal bars

Share other ideas with us on Facebook: **No Caffeine Required**.

Chapter 6: POWER Eating After Hours

Although this book is about food choices for the working week, it is also about making lifestyle habits that spill over into life outside the workplace. Whether you're staying in or eating out, you need to stay mindful of the POWER principles to keep yourself energised and feeling great. This chapter helps you continue the POWER Eating Programme™ seamlessly beyond the working day so wherever you are, you don't get caught out by the energy drainers.

Beat the after-work munchies

Your energy levels are bound to flag after a busy day at work but that doesn't mean you have to slump into an armchair for the rest of the evening. If you've eaten your mid afternoon snack you shouldn't feel ravenous when you get home so you can choose something nutritious (and delicious) rather than grabbing a beer and a bag of crisps. A glass of sparkling water with a dash of elderberry cordial or a slice of fresh lime with a few olives, roasted almonds and veggie sticks can be instantly revitalising.

Evening meals

Your evening meals should be no different from any other meals in terms of their 'balance of POWER' so ensure you eat well in the evening to enjoy plenty of energy the following day. There's obviously more scope to cook hot meals at home and there are some evening meal ideas in the Sample Weekly Meal Planner on page 57. Of course, any of the lunch suggestions can be eaten in the evening too, such as salads, soups or omelettes and a light meal is better than a heavy meal as you're more likely to get a better night's sleep.

Weekend planning

Whilst weekends are often a time to switch off from your working week, they can be hectic and your nutritional needs can easily fall by the wayside if you're rushing from pillar to post.

Planning is therefore still crucial to maximise your energy levels during your free time so make sure your nuts and seeds, fruit, oatcakes and water are always at hand.

One thing you can enjoy at the weekend that you won't have time for during the week is a protein-rich POWER brunch that will make you feel good all day. So go for a full English with lean bacon, organic sausage, grilled mushroom and tomatoes, or a mushroom omelette with a green leafy salad and toasted pumpkin seeds, or a slice of sourdough toast with hummus, avocado, turkey slices and cherry tomatoes.

Eating out

We are truly privileged to be surrounded by restaurants from all corners of the world and we may visit them at weekends, during the week or for a working lunch. Whatever the occasion, once you've grasped the principles of the POWER Eating Programme™, you will be able to choose perfectly balanced dishes that will make you feel great. Here are a few dishes from different types of cuisine that meet the POWER criteria perfectly:

Italian	
Choose	• Tricolore salad – mozzarella, avocado and tomato
	• Avocado with prawns
	• Spaghetti bolognaise - ask for less spaghetti and a side dish of energising vegetables
	• Roast duck leg with broccoli, asparagus, green beans and new potatoes
Avoid	• Pizza - contains too much dough
	• Garlic bread
	• Pasta carbonara – too much cream and pasta
	• Risotto – usually only rice and vegetables with no protein

Indian	
Choose	• Chicken tikka (dry roasted in oven) • Tandoori mixed grill with dhal and handful of basmati rice • Chickpea curry with plain basmati rice and vegetables • Saag paneer - spinach with cottage cheese (high in protein)
Avoid	• Prawn crackers, Naan, poppadoms • Deep fried bhajis and samosas • Creamy curries such as korma, passanda or masala

Chinese	
Choose	• Crab and corn soup • Steamed fish with steamed vegetables and plain rice • Szechuan prawns • Chicken chop suey (stir-fried chicken, veg and bean sprouts) • Tofu
Avoid	• Prawn crackers • Egg fried rice • Sweet and sour battered pork balls • Spring rolls

Not so fast!

Avoid the fast food chains at all costs. Burgers, chips, deep-fried chicken, battered fish can have a negative effect on your energy and long term health.

A few handy tips in the restaurant

- Don't be afraid to ask off menu
- Ask the waiter to remove the bread basket and ask for olives instead
- Go for a starter and main course and skip the dessert
- Order extra vegetables
- Avoid desserts unless it's a fruit salad
- Avoid coffee in the evening and go for a peppermint tea instead or a camomile to promote a good night's sleep

Alcohol

We have already seen the effects of alcohol so if you're in the habit of drinking a couple of glasses in the evening your energy levels could suffer the following day.

Challenge: try eliminating alcohol completely for two weeks and monitor how you feel in your food diary. My clients feel so much better when there's less alcohol in their system. While you don't need to ban it completely, cutting down to a couple of glasses no more than three times a week would go a long way towards regaining your energy and vitality.

Chapter 7: Boost the POWER, Bust the Stress

If you've got to the point where you've started to plan your meals and your cupboards and desk drawers are brimming with POWER foods, then well done, you've made a fantastic start and you should already be feeling more energised and mentally alert. You may also be noticing other health benefits like fewer headaches, better digestion and, really importantly, a better ability to deal with stress.

In fact, my clients frequently report feeling less stressed when they switch to the POWER way of eating. This makes sense because maintaining steady blood sugar levels keeps the body calm and balanced without the need for adrenaline to bail you out. Thus with lower amounts of stress hormones coursing through your body, you respond to a previously stressful situation much more calmly.

Case study:

Charlotte came to one of my health and nutrition programmes. She always felt stressed out and her work/life balance was totally out of kilter. She then started to eat differently and this is what she said:

"The programme has changed the way I eat for life. I'm pleased to have lost weight but the real benefit has been how I feel: I'm less stressed, my skin is clearer than it has been for 20 years, and I feel like I have the energy to enjoy life again – so much so that I've stopped working weekends and met someone lovely to spend my time with!"

Whilst changing what you eat can make a big difference to how you cope with stress, in order to enjoy maximum energy you need to change not only what you eat, but HOW you eat. As we have seen in the opening chapter, eating very quickly or skipping meals can create a state of stress in the body, and as stress is a massive consumer of energy this way of eating can wear you out.

Furthermore, food isn't the only solution for keeping you energised and I have included lots of tips on how to incorporate exercise into your busy day, including some chill time and also, how to get a good night's sleep.

In order to bust the stress it's also necessary to address your 'emotional diet' as negative thoughts and emotions can drain you just as much as eating the wrong kind of food.

Read on for practical ways in which you can boost the POWER and reduce the stress to keep your energy flowing.

POWER Eating

How often should I eat?

Eat every 3 to 4 hours to keep your blood sugar balanced and beat the slump. After your super sustaining breakfast you shouldn't need to refuel for at least three hours, although keep drinking your water and herbals to stay hydrated. If you go for longer than four hours without food though your blood sugar levels will dip and you may end up grabbing the wrong food - and too much of it.

But I often forget to eat ...

If you're the kind of person who goes for hours without eating as you're 'too busy to eat' then to kick start your new habit of eating more frequently, why not stick a post-it on your screen saying "Snack" or "Drink" or set a reminder on your phone. Anything that can stop your blood sugar plummeting will be helpful.

How much should I eat?

Your main meals should fit into your two hands cupped together which represents the approximate size of your stomach. Never overload your digestive system by eating too much as this is the sure way to fall into that afternoon slump. Take a look at the POWER plate on page 22 again to remind yourself of a perfectly balanced meal and remember to go easy on the starchy carbs as they will drain your energy if eaten in excess - not to mention increase your waistline!

How should I eat?

To allow for proper digestion you need to eat slowly, calmly and mindfully. If you're stressed, the body switches to 'fight or flight' mode and blood flow is diverted away from the stomach to the muscles so it can deal with the expected "emergency". This disrupts the digestive process and the proper absorption of nutrients from your food, and can also cause indigestion making you uncomfortable for the rest of the day. So if you're the type who wolfs down their sandwich in two minutes flat then you need to find ways to slow down and savour your food so you can stay on an even keel throughout the day. Here are some tips to help you:

- Chew, chew and chew again! Digestion starts in the mouth so chewing starts the process off very nicely. Chewing also helps you eat mindfully, rather than mindlessly, helping you to focus on your food rather than who's just sent you an email. Set yourself a goal of chewing the first ten mouthfuls 20 times. It not only slows you down but also gives your stomach the chance to let your brain know that you're full - so chewing prevents overeating too.

- Stay hydrated. Drinking plenty of water will ensure adequate delivery of nutrients to your brain, keeping your energy and concentration levels high. If dehydrated, your body and brain will start to slow down so try lemon, ginger or peppermint infusions for an instant natural pick-me up. If you're not used to drinking water, setting an alarm on your computer or mobile can get you into the habit. Keep a 2 litre water bottle on your desk and make sure it's empty by the end of the day.

- Eat your lunch, if possible, in a quiet room where there are no distractions.

- If you have no option but to eat 'al desko', switch off the screen and don't answer the phone – let your voicemail take over.

- Move the keyboard out of the way, bring in your own table mat and cutlery and turn your desk into a dining table for half an hour.

- Escape! Find a park bench nearby and enjoy some down time away from the workplace.

- Focus on different sensations as you eat your food – the smell, the taste, the textures, the colours. You can even close your eyes and visualise your food emitting wonderful waves of energy that will keep you awake, alert and focused for the rest of the day.

- To aid digestion, add a couple of teaspoons of apple cider vinegar to warm water and sip before your meal or use it in your salad dressing mixed with olive oil.

- End the meal with a peppermint tea - the perfect digestif!

- Supplement if necessary. Probiotics and digestive enzymes can help you get the most out of your POWER meals (see Resources on page 106).

Ways to boost energy without food

It's not only food that affects your energy levels. If you're sitting for hours in one place, feeling low, bored and frustrated, this will wear you out too so instead of going for food, here are some non-food activities you need to do to shake off the slump and energise your day.

Get moving!

Exercise boosts your metabolism, pumps up the production of 'feel good' endorphins, helps keep you calm and clear-headed, and relieves stress. Although you may feel tired at first if you're not used to it, studies show that the more you exercise the more energy you have. So if you do sit at your desk for hours on end, aim to get up every half hour, so your body doesn't think you're ready to slow down and go to sleep. Ideas to get you moving:

- Take a brisk walk outside for 5 minutes or walk around the office to stretch your limbs

- Go up and down the stairs a couple of times and avoid the lift as much as possible

- Keep fit while you sit. Try some 'deskercise' to keep you toned and alert while you work (e.g. http://deskercises.com). Just enough to get your heart rate up slightly without feeling uncomfortable.

- Join a local gym and get energised for the afternoon.

Organise and prioritise

Staring at a seemingly endless to-do list is enough to zap your energy before you've even started it, so prioritise the tasks that are essential and postpone or even delete the less important ones.

Breathe!

Deep breathing is one of the best ways to relieve stress in the body. This is because when you breathe deeply it sends a message to your brain to calm down and relax, lowering adrenaline levels in the body. The brain then sends this message to your body[3]. Breathing deeply oxygenates your brain, keeping you mentally alert. So if you're feeling stressed, or to avoid feeling stressed, practice this simple breathing exercise every day:

- To breathe fully, sit up straight and place your hands on your belly, directly above your belly button. Let the fingertips of both hands touch lightly. Exhale fully through your mouth. Breathe in deeply through your nose and into your belly, so

---

[3] Stress management. In JE Pizzorno Jr, MT Murray, eds., <u>Textbook of Natural Medicine</u>, 3rd ed., vol. 1, pp. 701–708. St. Louis: Churchill Livingstone.

that your fingertips spread an inch apart. Let your belly fill with air. Hold your breath for two to five counts, and then exhale slowly through your nose. Match the length of the inhale with the length of the exhale. Continue breathing in this manner for five to ten minutes (www.livestrong.com).

• Yoga. Deep breathing forms an integral part of yoga so if you can, find a yoga class to attend that will keep you calm, energised and in control.

A change is as good as a rest

• If you're feeling bored or frustrated with your work, a knee-jerk reaction may be to work your way through a biscuit barrel as a distraction, with disastrous effects on your energy. So find something else to do like tidy your desk, sort out your inbox, delete unwanted files – these can all be very therapeutic and help restore your energy.

• Or just take a break and step outside for some fresh air.

Quit smoking

I appreciate this is easier said than done but the most important thing you need to do before you quit is to balance your blood sugar which of course is exactly what the POWER Eating Programme™ is all about. It's well known that many people who give up smoking put on weight. This is because their body is no longer releasing sugar from its stores in response to the nicotine so it needs to get the energy from somewhere else – i.e. food. If your blood sugar is balanced it means your body is getting what it needs so not only will your cravings for sugar diminish but you'll find it easier to give up the cigarettes too.

Power naps

Studies have shown that a short nap in the afternoon of no more than 30 minutes can lower stress levels, boost productivity and concentration so this could be a huge benefit to your working day. If you have your own office that's perfect, otherwise you may have a dedicated quiet room at work where there's no disturbance. Alternatively, if you drive to work, you could have a quick nap in your car. To help you get to sleep wear earplugs or headphones and an eye mask to block out the light. You could listen to an app with soothing music, or do a guided meditation. Don't exceed 30 minutes as you may end up in a deep sleep from which you will awaken feeling groggy rather than re-energised.

Positive Mental Attitude

However well balanced your diet and exercise regime, poor emotional health can drain all your energy.

Waking up with a lot of worry on your mind, feeling unhappy, dreading the day ahead, feeling angry and resentful towards your boss or co-workers all cause stress, and much of your energy will be re-directed towards dealing with the stress before you've even got out of bed!

Just as you can choose between eating brown bread or white bread you can choose to have positive or negative thoughts. Thus if you choose to appreciate and cherish rather than dread and hate, you can halt the draining effect of negative, stressful thoughts and enjoy renewed mental and emotional energy. I'm not suggesting this can happen overnight but with self-awareness, perseverance and plenty of practice this could be one of the most important habits you've ever made. Here are some tips to help you make the switch from negative to positive:

- Resolve conflicts. Arrange to resolve any discord in your life as this can drain all your energy, however well balanced your diet and exercise regime. So if you're harbouring a grudge against someone at work, try talking to them to find a solution rather than bottling it up - if a niggle turns into deep resentment it can pull you right down to the bottom of the energy ladder.

- Think about what you've achieved at the end of the day rather than what went wrong.

- Banish "I can't" and think "I can" and "I will" instead. Express this out loud if necessary.

- Cognitive Behavioural Therapy (CBT) or finding a counsellor who can help you resolve these issues can ultimately be an energy-saving exercise, allowing you to spend your time and energy on the more productive, constructive areas of your life.

- Learn to practise meditation for 20 minutes per day.

A good night's sleep

If you haven't slept well everything feels so much worse and it becomes an ordeal to get through the day without stimulants. Tips for ensuring good quality sleep:

- Get to bed around 11 pm and definitely before midnight.

- Switch off the computer at least one hour before retiring as the blue light is designed to keep you awake.

- Steer clear of caffeine in the evening as it can stay in the body for up to 12 hours - so if you are going to have a caffeinated drink, have one late morning. Don't forget that chocolate contains caffeine so avoid this too as it can prevent sleep.

- Try a herbal tea such as camomile to help you relax.

- If you feel hungry in the evening, avoid sugary snacks and have an oatcake with nut butter instead.

- The amino acid tryptophan helps promote sleep and sources include turkey, cottage cheese and seeds. Lettuce and celery can help induce sleep too.

- Magnesium is known as nature's tranquiliser and a supplement (with calcium) can be useful.

- Herbal remedies containing valerian, hops and passiflora can be helpful.

Practice makes perfect

Practise new habits every day and when you feel yourself slipping back into unhelpful eating habits, ask yourself "Is this going to sustain me or drain me?" and imagine the consequence of your choice before you decide.

Support each other

- Buddy up with your co-workers and encourage each other to stick to the POWER Eating Programme™.

- Rota – designate each person in the office to bring in a particular food on a weekly basis e.g. herbal tea, oatcakes, nut butter, fruit.

- Put a pound in a charity box if you go off the rails.

- Tell us about other ways you have found to support each other at work.

Chapter 8: Recipes

Many of these recipes are so simple that they require no more than throwing a few ingredients together to give you a super nutritious POWER meal. I have included a small selection of recipes here but will be frequently updating my website with many more so visit **www.nocaffeinerequired.com** and like my Facebook page: **No Caffeine Required** for more delicious, exciting ideas.

Breakfasts

Muesli

The best mueslis are oat-based with plenty of nuts and seeds and very little dried fruit. Despite their wholesome-looking packaging, shop bought mueslis can still be packed with malted wheat flakes and dried fruit, making them very sugary. So it's much better to make your own and here's my recipe:

> *250g (8oz) rolled jumbo oats (preferably organic)*
> *Sunflower and pumpkin seeds (can be toasted in a pan for a few minutes to crisp them up)*
> *Chopped hazelnuts and flaked almonds for a natural supply of fibre and essential fatty acids*
> *Desiccated or strips of coconut*
> *Fresh fruit such as blueberries, raspberries, grated apple or pear to provide extra vitamins and anti-oxidants*
> *Milk or dairy-free (I like oat or coconut)*
> *Flaxseeds (ground)*

Mix all dry ingredients together and store in a large plastic container.

As it's best to store flaxseeds in the fridge, these can be added just before eating along with the milk and fresh fruit. This amount will last you a good week and as it's eaten cold, can be easily transported to work in a good quality container (see Resources on page 106).

Ring the changes and add any of the following flakes: barley, quinoa, buckwheat, millet, rice, rye.

Overnight Porridge Oats (serves 1)

This can be eaten either hot or cold and can be prepared the night before.

75g (3oz) jumbo rolled oats, preferably organic, not quick cooking
240ml (8 fl oz) milk or alternative (e.g. oat or coconut milk)
1/4 tsp. vanilla extract
1/4 tsp. cinnamon

- Mix all the ingredients together in a bowl (or container if transporting to work) and cover.
- Leave overnight in fridge or allow to soak for at least half an hour before eating or cooking (softer and easier to digest).
- Add berries / grated apple / chopped pear / chopped nuts.
- Eat cold or heat on the hob or in the microwave to make porridge, adding a little extra liquid if too stodgy.

Granola

Again, avoid the shop bought variety as it is packed with honey, syrup, sugar and bad fats, so it really isn't healthy at all. Maple syrup has some wonderful properties, or if you prefer you can use acacia honey or agave syrup.

300g whole rolled oats
30g desiccated coconut
100g chopped organic raw nuts e.g. cashews, pecans, walnuts,
almonds, hazelnuts
1 large pinch fine sea salt
60g raw seeds e.g. sunflower, pumpkin, sesame
125 ml apple juice
2 tbsp coconut oil, melted
½ tsp vanilla extract or almond extract
2-3 tablespoons maple syrup or acacia honey

- Preheat oven to 160ºC (320º F), gas mark 3.

- Combine oats, coconut, nuts, seeds, and salt in a large bowl.
- In a separate bowl, whisk together the maple syrup, apple juice, coconut oil, and vanilla extract.
- Stir the wet mixture in with the dry ingredients until the oats are thoroughly coated.
- Spread mixture evenly over large baking tray and bake for 20 minutes.
- Stir and toss the granola as best you can and return to the oven for 20 minutes more.
- Then stir again and bake for final 10-20 minutes.
- Your granola will be ready when it is light golden brown and crisp to taste.
- Remove from oven and allow to cool.

This granola can be kept in an airtight container in a cool, dry place for up to two weeks.

Quinoa porridge with chia seeds, pear and vanilla

For those of you who prefer a grain-free, gluten-free breakfast this is another delicious idea using the wonderful quinoa (pronounced keen-wah) which is actually a seed, rather than a whole grain, and contains all the amino acids that make up a complete protein. Due to its protein and fibre content, quinoa packs a fantastic nutritional punch, keeping you satisfied and energised. It also contains calcium, magnesium, iron and zinc as well as the B vitamins – all important for energy, vitality and reducing stress too. The grain has a fluffy texture and nutty taste and if it doesn't turn out perfectly the first time you cook it, don't give up as it's a very worthy member of your store cupboard.

The tiny chia seeds are a rich source of omega 3 essential fats and turn gelatinous when soaked. Again, don't be put off by this seed as it really is a powerhouse of energy.

This porridge could take you through to lunch time as it's packed with POWER ingredients.

¾ cup of quinoa washed
2 tbsp chia seeds
1 ½ cups of water (ideally filtered)
1 pear or other fresh fruit chopped
¾ cup of milk or dairy-free e.g. coconut, oat or almond
1-2 teaspoons of maple syrup / agave syrup / acacia honey
(optional)
1 teaspoon of cinnamon
1/4 teaspoon vanilla bean paste or extract

- Place the quinoa and chia seeds in a lidded saucepan, add the water and leave to soak for 10 minutes to allow the chia seeds to absorb the water.
- Add the chopped pear, goji berries, vanilla paste, cover and cook on a low heat for 15 mins.
- Just before serving add the milk, drizzle with syrup and sprinkle with cinnamon.
- This is also good served cold so you can take it to work.

How to cook the perfect quinoa

90g/3oz dry quinoa per person
180 ml / 6fl oz water with 2 tsp Marigold stock
(1:1½ ratio of quinoa to liquid prevents it going soggy)
- Rinse the quinoa in a sieve under cold running water first to remove the bitter coating then dry roast it in a heavy bottomed saucepan for a minute or two, stirring constantly.
- Add the liquid and stock and bring to the boil.
- Turn the heat down and simmer gently until the liquid has been absorbed (about 13 minutes).
- Drizzle some olive oil, season and 'fluff up' with a fork.

Coconut flapjacks

80g coconut oil with olive oil (try 50/50)
60g agave nectar and 50 g maple syrup / acacia honey
50g peanut butter, no added sugar
175g porridge oats
50g ground almonds
55g desiccated coconut (sugar free)

- Preheat oven to 180°C / 350°F / Gas mark 4.
- Grease a medium-sized square baking tray.
- Melt the oil in a large saucepan with the Sweet Freedom.
- Stir over a low heat until melted then stir in all the other ingredients and mix together well.
- Turn the mix into the baking tray and spread out evenly.
- Bake for 15 minutes, then remove from the oven and cut into squares (approx. 12).
- Leave in the tin until completely cool, then turn out.

Apple and almond muffins

170g (6oz) plain wholemeal or spelt flour
55g (2oz) ground almonds
1 tsp baking powder
1 tsp bicarbonate soda
70g (2½ oz) unsalted butter, soft
1 large egg, beaten
2 tbsp runny honey or agave syrup
150ml (5fl oz) milk or dairy alternative
2 small eating apples, cored
Pinch of cinnamon

- Preheat oven to 190ºC (375ºF), gas mark 5.
- Grate apples by hand or in a food processor, and set aside.
- Place flour, ground almonds, baking powder, bicarbonate of soda into a bowl.
- In a separate bowl lightly whisk the egg, butter and honey.
- Add egg mix to first bowl along with the milk, grated apple and cinnamon. Stir until you achieve a 'dropping' consistency, adding more milk if required.
- Dollop the mixture into muffin cases to 2/3 full.
- Bake 15-20 minutes, until risen and golden and let cool.

Breakfast cookies (makes approx. 14)

125g wholemeal or spelt flour
150g jumbo porridge oats
1/2 tsp bicarbonate soda
Pinch of sea salt
1/2 tsp ground cinnamon
4 tbsp maple syrup or agave nectar
1 large carrot or 2 medium-sized carrots, coarsely grated
100ml olive or coconut oil
100g chopped dried apricots (preferably organic unsulphured)
100g chopped nuts or seeds
Grated zest of 1 lemon (optional)

- Preheat oven to 180°C / 350°F / Gas 4.
- Add the flour, oats, baking soda and salt to a big bowl. Mix well so the baking soda and salt are evenly distributed. Add the remaining ingredients. Mix everything together.
- Scoop by the tablespoon and press into rounds on an oiled baking sheet. Tidy up the edges. You'll probably get about a dozen per tray. If you don't want two batches, just freeze the rest of the mix for another day.
- Bake for around 10-15 minutes until lightly golden. Flip the cookies over and return to oven for 3 more minutes to crisp up the bottoms.
- Once cooked, they store nicely for a week in an airtight container.

Pâtés & Dips

Hummus

1 tin chickpeas, drained and rinsed
1 cup tahini paste
2 garlic cloves
2 lemons juiced
½ tsp cumin
Salt to taste

- Drain and rinse the chickpeas, and place in pan with water barely covering. Bring to boil and simmer for a few minutes. Remove from heat and take a spoonful or two of the chickpeas out – reserve for garnish.
- Add tahini and garlic to the chickpeas and the water in the pan, and 'blitz' in blender to form a smooth and creamy paste.
- Add lemon juice, cumin and salt to taste and more water if required.
- Garnish with toasted pine nuts, chopped parsley and the reserved chickpeas.

For the best hummus - use dried chickpeas:

- Soak them overnight. Change the water the next day and add 1 tbsp bicarbonate of soda to the cooking water.
- Bring to the boil, skim and cook slowly until soft.
- Use some of the cooking liquid to make the hummus as with tinned chickpeas.

Smoked mackerel pâté

250g smoked mackerel, skin and bones removed, flaked
200g natural yoghurt / crème fraîche
1 lemon, zested (optional) and juiced
1-2 tbsp creamed horseradish, to taste
Any or all of these herbs: 2 tbsp parsley, chives, dill chopped

- Put the smoked mackerel, crème fraîche / yoghurt, lemon juice (and zest) in a food processor and whizz until blended.
- Stir in the herbs and horseradish. Chill until ready to serve.
- Serve on 3 Oatcakes or 1 Slice of toasted rye bread with salad.

Alternative: you can use smoked trout instead or mix with the smoked mackerel for a delicious blend.

Salads

Brown rice & lentil salad (serves 2)

175g (6oz) brown basmati rice
400g (14oz) tin lentils, rinsed or 300g (10oz) of cooked lentils,
drained
6 spring onions
1 red pepper – diced
Flat parsley
2 oz unsalted cashews

Dressing

6 fl oz olive oil
3 tbsp Tamari sauce
2 tbsp lemon juice
1 clove garlic crushed
Seasoning to taste

- Cook rice for 25 minutes until soft and leave to cool.
- Meanwhile chop the vegetables and prepare the dressing.
- Mix together and keep chilled until required.

Quinoa and mackerel salad (serves 2)

140g/5oz quinoa
2 smoked mackerel fillets cut into 1 inch (2.5 cm) pieces
4 cherry tomatoes, halved
6 cm cucumber, chopped
1 red pepper, chopped
Marinated artichoke hearts
Rocket

- Cook quinoa (see instructions on page 86) and leave to cool.
- Meanwhile prepare the vegetables.
- Mix together and keep chilled until required.
- Add the dressing just before you eat to prevent soggy rocket.

Oven-baked vegetable frittata (serves 2)

1 tbsp extra virgin olive / coconut oil
1 red onion, chopped
3 new potatoes, thinly sliced with skin on (optional)
1 red pepper, chopped
1 medium courgette, thinly sliced
2 handful of spinach leaves
2 tbsp frozen peas
6 eggs
1 tbsp yoghurt (optional)
A handful of chives and parsley, roughly chopped
Freshly ground black pepper and small pinch of Himalayan salt

- Lightly fry onion in olive or coconut oil.
- Par boil the potatoes for 5-6 minutes and drain.
- Add courgettes, pepper and potatoes to the pan and cook until soft and golden – add the peas for the last 3 minutes.
- Whisk the eggs with milk and yoghurt.
- Pour egg mixture over vegetables.
- Season, add chives and parsley and stir.
- Allow to cook gently until the bottom is set, then slip the pan under a medium grill to brown the top.
- Serve warm or cold and cut into wedges.

Wraps

Chicken and avocado POWER wrap (serves 1)

Bursting with colour, fibre, wholegrain, lean protein and a dash of healthy fat - this wrap will keep the hunger under control and provide loads of nutrition.

1 wholegrain tortilla wrap
¼ avocado mixed with tbsp hummus - used as healthy spread
1 generous handful of baby spinach
1 thinly sliced tomato and any other salad vegetables you enjoy
100g thinly sliced chicken breast (or turkey)
Black pepper to taste

Soups

Janet's Tomato and Butterbean Soup (serves 2)

This is one of the simplest soups to make and can be put together in minutes.

1 tbsp extra virgin olive oil
1 large onion, chopped
425g (15oz) tin chopped tomatoes
425g (15oz) tin or carton of butterbeans (rinsed and drained)
1 bay leaf
2 tsp Marigold stock

- In a pan gently fry the onion for a few minutes until soft and translucent.
- Add the tomatoes, butter beans and bay leaf.
- Add boiling water and stock to barely cover the other ingredients.
- Bring gently to the boil, turn down the heat, cover with lid and simmer for 10 minutes.
- Remove bay leaf and liquidise.
- Add tamari, Worcestershire sauce or tabasco for extra flavouring.

POWER dressings

Apple Cider Vinaigrette

You can double up on quantity as this lasts for several days in the fridge. You can use balsamic vinegar and the general rule is one part vinegar to 3 parts oil. You can also replace vinegar with juice of a lemon, so experiment with different options.

1 tbsp Dijon mustard
3 tbsp olive oil (or a blend of oils e.g. flax or avocado oil)
1 tbsp apple cider vinegar

Place in a jar and shake well.

Yoghurt "Mayonnaise"

1 tablespoon Dijon mustard
150g (5½ oz) pot of natural yogurt or crème fraiche
3 tablespoons olive oil
Black pepper, to taste

Shake all ingredients in a jar until smooth.

"Soyannaise"

150g (5½ oz) tofu, diced
3 tbsp olive oil
1-2 tbsp lemon juice
1 tsp mustard powder
1 tsp light clear honey (e.g. acacia)
70ml (2¼ fl oz) water
Pinch of sea salt and fresh black pepper

Place all ingredients in a food processor e.g. Vitamix, add the water and blend until smooth and creamy.

Smoothies

POWER smoothie (serves 2)

2 tbsp chia seeds – soaked overnight
1 tbsp coconut fat
2 tbsp almond butter
½ banana
Berries e.g. blueberries, strawberries, raspberries (frozen are fine)
Apple
Cup of water
Cup of almond or coconut milk unsweetened
Protein powder (optional) e.g. hemp, whey or pea protein (see Resources on page 106)

Whiz up ingredients in your smoothie maker / blender.

Green smoothie (serves 1)

½ organic cucumber
½ avocado
1 apple
1 tbsp chia seeds (pre-soaked for at least 15 minutes)
1 handful organic kale (use spinach, romaine lettuce, chard,
broccoli or 2 sticks of celery if you can't get organic kale)
1-2 glasses coconut water (unsweetened)
1 tbsp green powder or protein powder e.g. hemp, pea or whey (see
Resources on page 106)

Reproduced with kind permission of Amelia Freer www.freernutrition.com

Whiz everything up in a blender. Add more coconut or filtered water to reach desired consistency.

Snacks

Spicy Chickpea nuts

When roasted in a hot oven, the chickpeas become super crunchy and make a great snack. Cook for 30-45 minutes until crunchy. Worth the wait!

425g (15oz) can chickpeas, rinsed
1 tbsp extra-virgin olive oil
2 teaspoons ground cumin
1 teaspoon dried marjoram
1/4 teaspoon ground allspice
1/4 teaspoon salt

- Position rack in upper third of oven; preheat to 230°C, 450°F, Gas Mark 8.
- Blot chickpeas dry with kitchen paper and toss in a bowl with oil, cumin, marjoram, allspice and salt. Spread on a baking sheet. Bake, stirring once or twice, until browned and crunchy, 30-45 minutes. Allow to cool on the baking sheet for 15 minutes.

Trail mix

Rather than having the same nuts every day, buy a few different varieties then mix them together for a tasty trail mix. Aim for about 80% nuts and seeds and 20% fruit to keep blood sugar balanced. Try this mix:

Seeds: toasted pumpkin and sunflower
Nuts: hazelnuts, macadamia, walnuts, soy nuts, raw or lightly roasted almonds
Unsweetened coconut strips
Goji berries or small amount of dried fruit: raisins / chopped dates / chopped apricots /cranberries)

Go to **www.nocaffeinerequired.com** for more delicious recipes.

Conclusion: POWER Eating in a Nutshell

If the prospect of changing your eating habits was daunting when you first started to read this book, you should now be feeling confident that there's nothing complicated about eating well to boost your working day. You should also see that rather than restricting you, the POWER Eating Programme™ offers you a greater variety of tasty, nutritious options than you may have enjoyed before.

One step at a time

Rome wasn't built in a day so you don't have to clear out your cupboards and buy everything on the shopping list in one go. Start with the simple changes like stocking up on nuts, oatcakes and fruit for your snacks then begin to make a list of all the things you'll need for this plan to work for you. Read chapters 4 and 5 to remind you.

Summing up

Whilst there are certain foods and drinks you will either never eat or never give up entirely, you still need to abide by some golden rules in order to stay at the top of the energy ladder. Here's a quick roundup of the lessons learnt and some tips on how to stay on the POWER trail.

- Avoid the Energy Drainers: sugary cereals, white bread, bagels, crisps, fried foods, doughnuts and pastries, biscuits, cakes and confectionery

- Get used to reading food labels so you know what to pick up and what to discard.

- Avoid the 'value' meals which may be cheap but may be full of additives, salt, sugar and bad fats.

- Control the starchy carbs and choose low GL foods, i.e. foods that supply a steady supply of energy. Remember that grains and starches are turned into sugar in the body so too many can upset your blood sugar, resulting in an energy slump.

Observe the recommended amounts for potatoes, pasta, bread, rice, carrots, corn etc on page 31.

- Memorise the POWER acronym so you can easily assess the nutritional balance of your meals. Here's a reminder:

P Protein
O Oils and Fats
W Whole Grains and Starchy Veg
E Energising Vegetables and Fruit
R Revitalising drinks

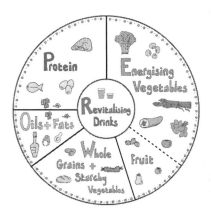

- Ask yourself "Where's my protein" with every meal including snacks, e.g. lean meat, beans, pulses, tofu, yoghurt, nuts and seeds. This helps keep your blood sugar balanced and prevents cravings and overeating. So even when you have an apple, eat a few almonds as well.

- Include plenty of 'good' fats from oily fish, nuts and seeds. Avoid the energy draining 'bad' fats found in margarine, fried foods, baked products and mayonnaise.

- Water water water! Keep a bottle of water with you at all times so that you're never dehydrated and you remain clear-headed and focused.

- Eat a 'rainbow' of vegetables every day.

- Include two portions of the less sugary fruits e.g. apples, pears, apricots and berries and avoid too much tropical fruit and grapes.

- Limit cups of coffee and tea to two per day. Reduce your caffeine intake slowly as sudden caffeine withdrawal can produce migraine-like symptoms for up to five days!

- Don't allow yourself to get hungry. Eat every three hours to avoid that blood sugar dip which can lead to low energy and cravings for the wrong kind of food

- Eat small portions so your brain doesn't need to divert all its energy to your stomach

- Plan meals in advance and ensure you are well stocked in all the things you need – look at the POWER meal solutions in Chapter 3 and the POWER staples on page 54 and make a list. Download the POWER shopping list from **www.nocaffeinerequired.com** to help you.

- Set aside some time to prepare your meals, even if it means putting a pot of nuts, seeds, an apple and a water bottle in your briefcase the night before.

- You don't need to make everything from scratch and provided you are discerning, you can find plenty of healthy options on the supermarket shelves.

- Chew your food well and eat mindfully, preferably away from your desk at lunchtime.

- Get up from your desk at regular intervals, preferably for two minutes every half an hour. (Study in American Journal of Clinical Nutrition 2013 showed that getting up two minutes every half an hour cut the risk of diabetes, lower blood sugar and insulin levels). Keep a schedule of activities to develop new habits.

- Breathe deeply to relieve the stress and take a break from email.

- Download the POWER Food and Energy diary and record your food intake and energy levels for a week. This is a very effective way of monitoring the effect of food on your energy levels. Complete the POWER checklist to ensure you're keeping on track.

- Re-do your **Health & Energy Monitor** every month to keep track of your energy and health improvements.

- Don't forget to visit **www.nocaffeinerequired.com** and sign up for the free newsletter and special offers.

- Fill in the feedback form and let us know how you're getting on.

I have enjoyed sharing my POWER secrets with you and hope you will be able to enjoy the same benefits as my other clients. Stay in touch and follow the POWER story on Facebook at **No Caffeine Required**. If you need help in implementing these tips then read on for the next steps ...

Here's to long lasting energy!

Next steps

Congratulations! Having read this book you now possess the tools and the 'POWER' to improve your energy levels and wellbeing, and hopefully you have already started to enjoy the benefits. In order to stay motivated and on track, there are a number of ways we can support you which are summarised below.

How we can support you

Food diary, plan and list

Go to **www.nocaffeinerequired.com** and download the POWER Food & Energy diary, Meal Planner and Shopping List. Don't forget to register for your FREE 5-day food diary analysis and meal plan - see details of bonuses on page iv.

Re-do the Health & Energy Monitor

It's easy to forget how you were feeling before you started the programme so fill in the Health & Energy Monitor again on page 102 and you should see a massive difference. Share your success with us on our **No Caffeine Required** Facebook page.

Seminars and workshops in the workplace

In order to help you and your colleagues implement the POWER Eating Programme™ at work, we can offer you a variety of seminars and workshops to suit your needs.

1. POWER @ Work Lunchtime Seminars (1 hour)
An informative and practical session, introducing you and your colleagues to the principles of the POWER Eating Programme™. This helps you make the best food choices to stay energised during your working day.

2. POWER Eating Workshops (3 hours)
An extension of the POWER @ Work Lunchtime Seminars, this is an informative, interactive and practical session helping you to

incorporate the POWER Eating Programme™ into your working day. Includes tips for planning your meals, recipes, recommended products and supplements, staying active every day, stress management & relaxation techniques.

3. Four-week Boost the POWER seminars (4 x 1-hour sessions)
An informative, motivational programme to help you and your colleagues consolidate the elements of the POWER Eating Programme™ over a 4-week period. Content similar to option 2 above and includes session on digestion and importance of exercise. Between sessions participants are advised to keep a food and energy diary on which they will receive feedback to ensure they are on track.

4. Online Food & Energy Diary Feedback (post-programme)
After attending any of the above workshops, or after reading this book, you and your colleagues can sign up for food diary analysis and support to help you cement what you've learnt on the programmes as well as keeping you motivated and on track. It is recommended that you keep a diary for at least one month to establish good habits.

5. Six-Week Zest4life Health & Weight loss Programme
Why go to a weight loss club when we can come along to you? As qualified Zest4life practitioners we can offer this weight management programme to you and your colleagues in the workplace to help you achieve your health and weight loss goals.

6. Private consultations
We also offer private consultations of 30 or 60 minutes either in the workplace or by telephone.

See **www.nocaffeinerequired.com** and contact us for further details.

Health and Energy Monitor (after 4 weeks)

You may have been shocked by your score when you first completed the Health and Energy Monitor (see page v). After four weeks of following the programme, fill in the form again and compare your scores with the original – hopefully you'll have something to celebrate!

How are you feeling?

Disagree .... Agree

I feel tired most of the time	1	2	3	4	5
I have poor memory / concentration	1	2	3	4	5
I am often stressed / anxious	1	2	3	4	5
I am prone to colds, flu, infections	1	2	3	4	5
I am overweight	1	2	3	4	5
I often have mood swings	1	2	3	4	5
I am prone to hormonal symptoms	1	2	3	4	5
I am prone to headaches	1	2	3	4	5
I don't sleep well	1	2	3	4	5
I suffer from indigestion / bloating	1	2	3	4	5
I am often constipated	1	2	3	4	5

Your total score: [ ]   Ideal score: 14 or less

How's your energy / blood sugar?

Disagree .... Agree

I need coffee, tea or something sweet to get me going in the morning	1	2	3	4	5
I have less energy than I used to	1	2	3	4	5
I feel tired 20 minutes after getting up	1	2	3	4	5
I often crave sweet foods, bread, chocolate, cereal, pasta	1	2	3	4	5
I often have energy slumps during the day	1	2	3	4	5
I often crave a coffee / something sweet after meals	1	2	3	4	5
I often overreact to stress	1	2	3	4	5
I find it difficult to concentrate at work	1	2	3	4	5
I often feel too tired to exercise	1	2	3	4	5
I am gaining / finding it hard to lose weight	1	2	3	4	5

Your total score: [ ]   Ideal score: 12 or less

The Glycemic Index & Load of Common Foods

Food	GI	GL	Serving size (g or ml)
Bread, baked goods			
Baguette, white	95	14	30
White wheat bread	73	11	30
Whole wheat bread	68	7	30
Pizza, cheese	60	16	30
Pitta bread, white	57	10	30
Pitta, whole wheat	56	8	30
Sourdough wheat bread	54	8	30
Sourdough rye bread	48	6	30
Pasta, rice, grains			
Sushi rice	85	33	150
White rice	73	30	150
Brown rice	66	22	150
Long grain rice	56	24	150
Basmati, white	57	23	150
Couscous	69	23	150
Buckwheat noodles	58	25	150
Quinoa	53	13	150
Sweet corn, canned	46	13	150
Spaghetti, white	42	20	180
Spaghetti, whole wheat	42	17	180
Barley, hulled, boiled	22	9	150
Breakfast cereals			
Kellogg's cornflakes	93	23	30
Kellogg's Rice Krispies	82	22	30
Instant oat porridge	83	18	250
Kellogg's Special K	69	14	30
Porridge, rolled oats	42	9	250
Muesli (Alpen), no sugar	59	11	30
Oats, raw	59	11	30
Fruit, fresh, canned and dried (values vary according to degree of ripeness)			
Banana, raw	42-62	11-16	120
Dates, dried	31-62	14-21	60

Food	GI	GL	Serving size (g or ml)
Cherries, raw	63	9	120
Mango, raw	41-60	9	120
Pineapple, raw	51-66	6-8	120
Grapes, black	59	11	120
Raisins, dried	66	28	60
Apricot, raw	34-57	3-5	120
Apricot, dried	30	8	60
Apple, raw	28-44	4-6	120
Pear, raw	34-42	4-5	120
Watermelon, raw	72-80	4-5	120
Orange, raw	31-51	3-6	120
Peach, raw	28-56	4-5	120
Plum, raw	25-53	3-6	120
Prunes, dried	29	10	60
Blueberries, raw	54	5	120
Strawberries, raw	40	1	120
Dairy products and non-dairy alternatives			
Soy milk, plain, unsweetened	44	8	250
Rice milk	79-92	17-29	250
Yoghurt, plain, fat-free	35	12	200
Yoghurt, strawberry, fat-free	61	18	200
Ice cream, chocolate	68	10	50
Beans and legumes (pulses)			
Red kidney beans, boiled	51	12	150
Baked beans, canned	40	6	150
Navy/haricot beans, boiled	31	9	150
Chickpeas, boiled	31	9	150
Black beans, boiled	30	7	150
Lentils, green, boiled	22	1	150
Lentils, red, boiled	18-31	3-6	150
Soy beans, boiled	15	1	150
Hummus (chickpea dip)	6	0	30
Starchy vegetables			
Instant mashed potato	97	19	150
Potato, white, boiled	96	24	150

Food	GI	GL	Serving size (g or ml)
Potato, baked, with skin	69	19	150
Mashed potato	83	17	150
Beetroot, boiled	64	4	80
French fries	64	21	150
Carrots, raw	16	8	80
Carrots, cooked	33-49	2	80
Sweet potato, boiled	44	11	150
Pumpkin, butternut, boiled	51	3	80
Drinks			
Fanta	68	23	250
Beer	66	5	250
Coca cola	63	16	250
Lemonade	54	15	250
Orange juice	46	12	250
Apple juice	44	13	250
Carrot juice	43	10	250
Snacks			
Mars bar	68	27	60
Snickers bar	68	23	60
Potato crisps	60	12	50
Twix bar	44	17	60
Plain milk chocolate	49	14	50
Dark chocolate	23	6	50
Tortilla chips	72	21	50
Sweeteners			
Glucose	100	10	10
Sucrose (table sugar)	60	6	10
Honey	35-87	6-18	10
Acacia honey	32	7	20
Fructose	11	1	10
Agave syrup	11	1	10

Resources

Supplements

There are many companies that produce good quality supplements e.g. Biocare, Viridian, Lamberts, Solgar amongst many others) and I recommend you buy them from your local health store or order online:

The Natural Dispensary 01453 757792
www.naturaldispensary.co.uk (Bonus: go to
www.nocaffeinerequired.com for 10% discount)

Totally Nourish 0800 085 7749 **www.totallynourish.com**

Bee Prepared Daily Defence or Max Strength contain bee propolis, black elderberry, olive leaf and beta glucans to support your immune system and help keep the bugs away. Available from The Natural Dispensary (above), health food stores or **www.unbeelievablehealth.co.uk.**

Green powders

E.g. Nutricology Progreens or Synergy Organic Supergreens.

Protein powders

E.g. Solgar Whey to Go or Pulsin' Pea Protein

Energy bars and cereals

Protein bars e.g. Bounce, Pulsin', Nakd – available from health food stores, selected supermarkets and The Natural Dispensary (above).

Lizi's Granola is a low-GL granola available from most supermarkets, health food stores and from **www.lizis.co.uk.**

Coconut oil

Coconoil – high quality organic extra virgin coconut oil available from many health food stores and from **www.coconoil.co.uk**

Instant veg pots

The Food Doctor www.thefooddoctor.com
Innocent **www.innocentdrinks.com** - Indian dahl curry lowest in sugar Available from health food stores and most supermarkets

Containers

A wide variety of Bpa-free bottles, flasks and containers are available to order e.g. from Amazon or Lakeland **www.lakeland.co.uk**.

Organic food box deliveries

Abel & Cole www.abelandcole.co.uk
Riverford www.riverford.co.uk

Seed sprouters

Biosnacky **www.avogel.co.uk/sprouts-biosnacky** available from good health food shops

Vitamix

Powerful blender for making smoothies, soups, nut butters Department stores e.g. John Lewis, Selfridges and Amazon www.vitamix.co.uk

Zest4life Nutrition & Weight Loss Programmes

A health and nutrition club based on low-GL principles that provides advice, coaching and support for losing weight and gaining health through a series of weekly meetings. For more information visit www.zest4life.com or email Lindamunster@zest4life.eu

Recommended books

Briffa, John. *Escape the Diet Trap*, Fourth Estate (2013)
Erasmus, Udo. *Fats that Heal, Fats that Kill*, Alive Books
(1993)
Holford, Patrick. *The Low-GL Diet Bible*, Piatkus (2009)
Holford P. & Mcdonald Joyce F: The *Holford Low-GL Diet
Cookbook*, Piatkus (2005)
Lustig, Robert. *Fat Chance: The Bitter Truth about Sugar*,
Fourth Estate (2013)
Marber, Ian. *The Food Doctor Everyday Diet*, Dorling
Kindersley (2005)

Websites:

www.patrickholford.com – information on health and
nutrition, health advice and products
www.drbriffa.com - a health-focused blog by British doctor
offering evidence-based, trustworthy and practical advice on
all aspects of healthy living
www.mercola.com - a reliable source of health articles,
optimal wellness products, medical news, and free natural
newsletter from natural health expert Dr. Joseph Mercola

Glossary

ATP

Adenosine triphosphate (ATP) is known as the 'energy currency' of all living cells. It is the molecule that stores the energy we need to do just about everything we do and is manufactured in tiny energy factories called mitochondria.

Free radicals

These are unstable molecules that can cause a lot of damage in the body if left unchecked. Whilst small amounts are helpful in everyday metabolic processes, too many can result in accelerated ageing and disease. Free radicals can be produced in vast quantities as a result of stress, too much sun, burnt or barbecued foods, smoking, bad food and drink habits and stress. Ultimately, they attack our cells draining them of energy and life.

Antioxidants

These are the antidote to free radicals, which are also known as oxidants, as they mop them up and protect our cells from damage. Antioxidants are abundant in fruit and vegetables, protecting us from disease and helping to slow down the ageing process.

Adrenals

The adrenal glands are situated above the kidneys and are each approximately the size of a walnut. They are mainly responsible for producing adrenaline and cortisol in response to stress. Continuous production of these stress hormones, coupled with inadequate rest, eventually wears out our system, making it difficult to cope with stress. This is known as "adrenal fatigue" or burnout.

About the Author

Linda Munster is an experienced nutrition consultant, having studied for four years at the renowned Institute for Optimum Nutrition. Since 2008 she has run a successful private practice and helped many clients with a range of health issues. She runs public courses on Nutrition and Weight Loss and her POWER @ Work seminars and workshops have been well received in the workplace.

Before studying nutrition Linda spent over 12 years delivering training to corporate staff in financial institutions both in Europe and the UK.

She now lives in north-west London with her husband and two grown-up children.

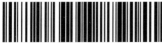

Made in the USA
Lexington, KY
17 February 2015